SUMMARY OF DENTAL ASSISTING NATIONAL BOARD (DANB) ELIGIBILITY PATHWAYS FOR THE CERTIFIED DENTAL ASSISTING (CDA) EXAM AND GENERAL CHAIRSIDE COMPONENT EXAM*

Pathway I:

1. Graduation from a CODA-accredited dental assisting or dental hygiene program
   AND
2. Current CPR from a DANB-accepted provider

Pathway II:

1. High school graduation or equivalent
   AND
2. Minimum of 3,500 hours of approved work experience
   AND
3. Current CPR from a DANB-accepted provider

Pathway III:

1. Former DANB CDA status, or graduation from a CODA-accredited DDS or DMD program, or graduation from a dental degree program outside the U.S. or Canada
   AND
2. Current CPR from a DANB-accepted provider

★There are no prerequisites to take DANB's Radiation Health and Safety (RHS) or Infection Control exams (ICE).

From website of Dental Assisting National Board, Inc. Chicago: www.danb.org. Accessed October 1, 2015. *Eligibility pathways subject to change annually.* DANB, CDA, RHS, and ICE are registered trademarks of the Dental Assisting National Board, Inc. (DANB). This publication and its companion website are not reviewed or endorsed by DANB.

MOSBY
REVIEW
QUESTIONS AND ANSWERS
FOR DENTAL
ASSISTING

SECOND EDITION

REVISED REPRINT

Edited and contributed by

**Betty Ladley Finkbeiner,
CDA–Emeritus, BS, MS**

Emeritus Faculty
Washtenaw Community College
Ann Arbor, Michigan

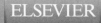

3251 Riverport Lane
St. Louis, Missouri 63043

REVIEW QUESTIONS AND ANSWERS FOR DENTAL ASSISTING,
SECOND EDITION (REVISED REPRINT)   ISBN: 978-0-323-44491-0

ISBN: 978-0-323-44491-0

Acquisitions Editor: Kristin Hebberd
Developmental Editor: Joslyn Dumas
Publishing Services Manager: Julie Eddy
Senior Project Manager: Andrea Campbell
Design Direction: Jessica Williams

Printed in the United States of America

Last digit is the print number: 9 8 7 6 5 4 3 2 1

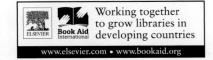

Reviewers and Contributors

Emily L. Addison, CDA, BS
Director of Dental Assisting
Pearl River Community College
Hattiesburg, Mississippi

Carol Ann Chapman, CDA, RDH, MS
Dental Clinical Associate
Dental Hygiene Program
Edison State College
Fort Myers, Florida

Jamie Collins, CDA, RDH
Dental Assisting Instructor
College of Western Idaho
Eagle, Idaho

Sharron J. Cook, CDA
Program Director and Instructor
Dental Assisting Program
Columbus Technical College
Columbus, Georgia

W. Stephan Eakle, DDS
Professor, Clinical Dentistry
Emeritus Division of General Dentistry
Department of Preventive & Restorative Dental
    Sciences
School of Dentistry
University of California, San Francisco
San Francisco, California

Aimee Marie Gaspari, BS, EFDA
Dental Assisting Instructor
YTI Career Institute
Lancaster, Pennsylvania

Cynthia Porter Giles, CDA, EFDA, PhD
Dental Coordinator
Centura College–Norfolk
Norfolk, Virginia

Mary Govoni, RDA, RDH, MBA
Speaker, Author, Consultant
OSHA/HIPAA Compliance and Health Care
    Ergonomics
Mary Govoni & Associates
Okemos, Michigan

Laura Howerton, RDH, MS
Instructor, Dental Hygiene
Wake Technical Community College
Raleigh, North Carolina

Teresa Macauley, CDA, EFDA, MS
Professor and Chair
Dental Assisting Program
Ivy Tech Community College
Anderson, Indiana

Chris H. Miller, MS, PhD
Professor Emeritus of Oral Microbiology
Executive Associate Dean Emeritus
Associate Dean Emeritus for Academic Affairs
    and Graduate Education
School of Dentistry
Indiana University
Indianapolis, Indiana

Linda Lee Paquette, RDA, CDA, RDH, MS
Faculty
Dental Assisting and Dental Hygiene Programs
Department of Health Sciences
Santa Rosa Junior College
Santa Rosa, California

Jennifer L. Poovey, CDA, RDA, RDH, BS
Faculty
Dental Assisting and Dental Hygiene Programs
Department of Health Sciences
Santa Rosa Junior College
Santa Rosa, California

Kathy Zwieg, LDA, CDA
Associate Publisher and Editor-in-Chief
Inside Dental Assisting
AEGIS Publications;
Executive Committee and Board Member
Oral Health America
Lino Lakes, Minnesota

Preface

The purpose of this book is to provide a steadfast review for the dental assisting student preparing for course review, local or state exams, or national certification. Three comprehensive tests are included in the format, all common to national exams for dental assistants. Tests are divided into the following categories:

- General Chairside (360 questions total/120 questions per test)
- Radiation Health and Safety (300 questions total/100 questions per test)
- Infection Control (300 questions total/100 questions per test)

For added convenience, each question is repeated in the answer key with the rationale for the correct choice so the results can be checked.

The companion Evolve website will allow you to test yourself electronically and includes an additional 640 practice questions (the equivalent of two full national board–style exams) with an additional 500 questions devoted specifically to expanded functions in dental assisting, divided by both topic and states in which they are approved for practice.

ABOUT THE EVOLVE WEBSITE

The companion Evolve website provides more opportunities to review specific topics. All 960 questions in the book plus an additional 640 questions (1,600 total) are available electronically; this is the equivalent of five full national board–style exams. The program lets you choose to practice in one of two ways: (1) in practice mode or (2) in exam mode.

In practice mode, you can choose the overall topic (General Chairside, Radiation Health and Safety, or Infection Control) as well as the subtopics into which those categories are divided (e.g., "Collection and Recording of Clinical Data" or "Chairside Dental Procedures" within the General Chairside exam), as well as how many questions you want to practice of the total provided. For instance, the database of questions for the Infection Control exam contains 50 questions on the topic of "Patient and Health Care Worker Education," and you can choose to practice from 1 to 50 questions in this category. Questions are randomized from each test so you will not necessarily see the questions in the same order in which they appear in the book. Immediate feedback is given after an answer is selected.

In exam mode, you can choose to have the site's test generator auto-create a simulated exam from the bank of 1,600 questions; this exam would match the number and distribution of questions per category within the CDA exam to provide targeted preparation and help build your confidence. A test timer is included to help you manage your test-taking time allotment, and feedback is provided after you complete the exam to easily show you where your strengths and weaknesses lie.

In addition, the website includes a separate section of 500 questions on a variety of expanded functions in dental assisting. Questions can be selected by topic or by state. If you choose the state option, the program will randomize questions for each topic approved for practice in the state selected.

EXPANDED FUNCTIONS IN DENTAL ASSISTING

It should be noted that expanded functions (EF) vary by state. The EF questions that are included have not been written for any particular location. We urge all users of this product to be familiar with the current approved EF for their states by contacting the appropriate boards of dentistry or other governing agencies.

Preparing for a Credentialing Examination—Guidelines for the Candidate

Betty Ladley Finkbeiner

As you open this book, you may be asking yourself, "Why am I doing this?" You may think, "I don't need to do this to have a job as a dental assistant." That may be true in some situations, but in many regions of the country you need a validated standard of performance in accordance with state dental laws. However, there are many reasons that you should have a professional credential. Anyone who tells you otherwise is not thinking about your professional worth or the importance of such a credential to your patients.

The first and foremost reason for a credential is to practice legally. As a dental assistant, you should be familiar with the dental law within the state in which you are employed. Many states require documentation of a professional credential to prove your performance in one or more areas of dental assisting. A list of national organizations and contacts for each state's board of examiners is included in the back of this book.

Patients who are in the care of a licensed dentist expect the dentist to employ qualified personnel. Further, they should expect that each of these employees will have completed all of the necessary education and, where applicable, secured a professional credential. By obtaining a recognized professional credential in dentistry, you have proven that you have the minimal qualifications to practice the duties that are legally delegable in your state. The credential should be posted where patients can visibly recognize your professional status.

By completing the Dental Assisting National Board (DANB) Certified Dental Assistant (CDA®) Infection Control or Radiography examination, you

have validated that you are familiar with the basic concepts of a technical, safe practice. This is important to your employer and to the patients who come under your care. Today's patients are concerned with their safety and are aware of potential hazards that exist in health care. You can allay some of their fears if you demonstrate knowledge in the areas of infection control, radiography, and quality assurance. Further, putting into practice these concepts and the appropriate guidelines from various governing agencies can only serve to protect you, the dental staff, and the patients.

Finally, having a credential that recognizes your knowledge and skills can only serve to increase your self-esteem. For some, this is most important because it shows that you have a documented base of knowledge that is recognized by the dental profession and you have become an important member of the dental health team....it could also result in a salary increase.

GETTING READY

What is the most important thing a student should do to prepare for an exam?

a. Get a good night's sleep before the exam and eat only a light breakfast.
b. Take two aspirin or ibuprofen before entering the exam room to ward off the distraction of a possible headache.
c. Develop a positive attitude of cautious optimism—that is, "I know I will pass this exam."
d. Develop a thorough understanding of the body of knowledge and concepts to be covered by the exam.

If you chose "d," you are off to a good start in preparing yourself for any exam, particularly those like the DANB or the state board credentialing exams. There is only one way to conquer a well-developed exam—to know the answers to the questions. The "trick" to obtaining good test scores is primarily to retain and apply the knowledge and skills learned in formal course work and in clinical applications. Various ways of helping you develop this strategy will be discussed later.

If you selected "c," you chose an important response but not the "best" one. It *is* important to go into any exam with a positive attitude and minimal anxiety, but such an attitude is realistic only if you do have a good command of the subject.

If you chose "a," then perhaps you interpreted the words "prepare for an exam" to mean only those things that should be done on the day before and the day of an exam. But preparation for an exam begins on the day you learn the first vocabulary word or the first concept associated with any area of learning. Exams are just one phase in the total ongoing learning process.

Answer "b" in the opening example is not a suitable response. It should be obvious that aspirin, ibuprofen, or any other drug cannot compensate for knowledge.

Before beginning to study for any type of exam, there are at least three things to do: (1) Secure a set of objectives for the area or areas that the examination is designed to evaluate, (2) secure a set of sample questions that are similar to the ones to be used on the examination for which you will be studying, and (3) review the materials in 1 and 2 thoroughly.

LEARNING ABOUT THE EXAMINATION

Whether you are preparing for a national certification examination such as the DANB or a state board or regional credentialing exam you need to be familiar with the material that will be covered. During the application process, you will be provided with an outline of the content and rules to follow on exam day. Pay close attention to the content outline and to the number of questions to be asked on each topic. (For information about the DANB exam, visit the website at www.danb.org and click on the DANB Exam button on the left.)

If you are taking a state board or regional exam that includes a clinical component, thoroughly review the list of materials you are to bring. If a patient is part of the clinical component, review the clinical requirements of the patient to ensure that your patient meets the criteria for the exam procedure. You should become familiar with the patient before the exam and not be forced to work with an unfamiliar patient. Do not wait until the day before the test to prepare your clinical tray or box because you may find that you do not have access to some material or instrument and may need to buy or borrow some device.

EXAMINATION FORMAT

In addition to knowing the content to be covered, it is important to know that written exams are usually multiple choice. All questions are apt to be in that format, with one best answer for each question. Many multiple choice questions are written with distracters (responses that are not the answers) that are partially correct or that are correct but not the best answer.

Some critics of multiple choice tests claim that you can score well on such a test by memorizing facts and learning some tricks to answering these types of questions. Such criticism is not true for any well-developed national or state credentialing exam. The test you take will have been prepared by test specialists. Each test question will have been tried out in regular testing situations with students in classes for dental assistants. You will be taking a great risk if you assume that skillful "guessing" will produce a passing score.

No written exam can test your ability to apply the knowledge or the understanding that you must possess to function as a dental assistant. Some state credentialing exams are apt to include a practical or clinical test, a test in which you will be asked to "demonstrate" what you have learned by doing such things as producing a full crown or intracoronal interim restoration or placing a rubber dam. Any of the clinical tasks, especially expanded functions that you have learned to do, may serve as a "situational" test in which your actual performance is observed and graded. It provides final evidence of whether a candidate can "put it all together" and function satisfactorily in a setting that simulates real life in a dental office.

When planning to take a practical clinical exam, you must prepare yourself to provide a variety of armamentarium. You will likely be required to provide a patient on whom to perform a given task, provide instruments, and sometimes purchase a model or two on which you may perform a specific task. In such cases, you should read the application thoroughly and understand the preparation long before the exam. In fact, it is wise to read over the list of materials and the patient requirements more than once to be certain you have not overlooked an item or a certain criterion for the patient. These materials should be obtained long before the exam and prepared in a container for transporting them safely to the exam. Avoid storing the materials in your vehicle because temperatures in some zones may alter the setting time of many dental materials you need to provide. Do not wait until the last week to prepare for such an exam because you may find yourself unable to obtain these materials at the last minute.

The purpose of any credentialing exam is to determine the extent to which each candidate has mastered the knowledge, concepts, and skills necessary to perform satisfactorily as a dental assistant. No exam, either written or practical, can be long enough to actually cover every concept or skill. Therefore, test developers must select questions and practical situations that are typical of the total body of knowledge and skills in dental assisting. As a candidate, you will not know what specific concepts and skills you will be tested on. The only solution is to be well prepared in all aspects of dental assisting.

For written exams, the multiple choice questions are considered the most versatile. They are a good method for measuring the knowledge of technical vocabulary and specific information that dental assistants must possess. They are also an effective method of measuring your understanding of relationships and interrelationships (whether things go together). It may be used for measuring your application of knowledge to situations that are different from ones you may have experienced previously.

About the only type of cognitive skill that is *not* measured well by multiple choice questions is creativity. Although credentialing exams are designed to find out whether you have mastered the basic fundamental skills of a subject area, they are not designed to discover potential talent for creative innovations.

On any certification, registry, or licensure exam, you will be tested on how well you have acquired and internalized the basic language, concepts, and skills of dental assisting—the things that must become second nature to you as a practicing dental assistant.

STUDYING

The best preparation for a credentialing exam is to be prepared for every dental assisting class that you take. The required textbooks for courses in dental assisting should be studied carefully, not only for immediate acquisition of knowledge, but particularly for internalization and retention of that knowledge. Many students find it helpful to highlight key passages in a text so they can go back and skim those

passages easily. This same marking system also works if you have taken online courses and have downloaded lectures. Sometimes the author(s) of a text will emphasize important points for you by paragraph headings or by italicized sentences. Acquisition and retention of important concepts require repetition for most people. Therefore, taking the time during an initial reading to make review work easy is time well spent.

Taking good class notes is a very important study skill. Many instructors spend some time making key points and quite a lot of time illustrating these points. Most students are well advised to concentrate on writing down the key points without trying to take notes verbatim. It may be helpful to write down some of your instructor's examples, but only if these examples seem necessary to remember the discussion. If the instructor provides outlines or copies of PowerPoint slide presentations, use a colored marker to highlight important points.

Some students find it difficult to review their own notes after a lecture. It is wise to date the notes, make a heading title on the page, review the notes as soon as possible, and, when necessary, recopy the notes for better understanding. If after you have reviewed and edited your notes you have doubts about a concept or basic information, be sure to ask your instructor for clarification as soon as possible.

In addition to identifying the key concepts from text materials, lectures, and notes, it is important to develop a thorough understanding of the dental vocabulary. Every profession has its own vocabulary—not only the technical words that identify important materials, concepts, rules, and ideas—but also the words commonly used to communicate in the profession. Technical vocabulary will be tested in any written or practical exam. In addition, the questions that you will be asked on any credentialing exam will be worded in the day-to-day language of the profession. To progress through the test efficiently, it is essential that you understand quickly and completely each question that you are asked. If you do not understand a question, it will be difficult to answer it correctly.

In addition to the general suggestions for learning and studying throughout your education, there are other options that may be helpful as you review material in preparation for a credentialing exam. Some schools provide review sessions or classes to prepare you. However, if these are not available, one of the most effective steps you can take is to develop cooperative study sessions with one or two friends.

Such sessions are best conducted as much like a classroom situation as possible; that is, each person should develop a series of questions to ask the other(s) along with the materials necessary to answer the questions before the joint study session. If your colleagues miss any of the questions, you should be prepared to explain the answer to them and vice versa. Teaching a concept or skill to someone else is one of the best learning techniques to acquire familiarity with that concept or skill yourself. Consequently, your weakest area is the best one to teach to others. Naturally, study sessions such as these are not comparable with a formal class, but they should be conducted in a businesslike fashion. If these study sessions become just a social outing among friends, you may enjoy them, but they will cease to contribute much to your exam preparation.

Regardless of whether you take a formal review class or develop a study session with colleagues, such an experience will likely be very beneficial. A bonus of these sessions is enhanced confidence in your ability to do well on an exam. Nothing builds confidence as much as feeling that you have mastered some area of knowledge or skill so well that you can help others understand it as well.

FRAME OF MIND

It is wise and prudent to prepare yourself physically for an exam by getting at least 8 hours of sleep and avoiding caffeine. Keep in mind that the test you are taking in dental assisting is to measure your mental abilities and not your physical prowess. Studying all night before an exam is not a recommended behavior. Physical fatigue can depress test-taking efficiency. The best physical preparation is simply to avoid any major variation from your normal routine.

Preparing for a good mental attitude means that you develop confidence that you have adequately prepared yourself and that you expect to do well. You may approach an exam with some degree of anxiety, like an athlete who enters a competition. This feeling is not necessarily bad. Research indicates that some test anxiety, as long as it is not severe, may help to produce a positive result.

There is a myth that large numbers of students "clutch" when taking exams, particularly written exams. No doubt there are some individuals who have developed psychological blocks to taking tests, but from my teaching experience, I have noted that many (probably most) students who claim that a low test score was caused by an inability to perform well

on tests have not developed the requisite knowledge and skills to answer the questions.

Sometimes repeated practice on similar written exams will be helpful. But if you feel you have a serious test-taking problem, it may be necessary to seek some professional counseling to overcome this situation. Some of the following suggestions may help if you have difficulty taking tests.

- Bring all of the necessary admission and testing materials with you. Follow the guidelines provided for you by the testing agency.
- When entering the testing room, choose a seat that will be comfortable for you, unless you are assigned a seat or location.
- Read carefully the printed directions given to you.
- Listen carefully to the verbal directions. Do not assume that because you have taken many exams that the directions will be the same for this one.
- If the directions are not completely clear to you, ask the examiner in charge of the session to explain exactly what is required.
- Understand completely the mechanics that you are expected to follow during the exam.
- In a written test, you will be given multiple choice questions in a booklet and a separate answer sheet.
  - Do not make responses hurriedly or carelessly.
  - Be certain you place your answer on the correct form, on the correct line, and in the space provided.
- On a computer test, you will enter your answers on the screen.
  - Be certain that your selection is placed in the correct space provided.
- Be cautious when you correct an answer that your previous answer has either been erased or deleted in either the paper or computer testing format.
- Be certain to answer every question.
  - Most computer test formats will alert you if you have not answered specific questions and you can then scroll back to these questions.
  - In a written format, you will need to review your answer sheet for blank spaces to ensure that you have entered an answer for every question.
  - You must arrive at one correct or one "best" answer.
  - If you must, "guess" between two alternatives or eliminate the two or three answers you know are wrong first.

- If you can eliminate any responses as incorrect based on your knowledge, you will not be guessing randomly but will be exercising "informed guessing."
- In a clinical exam, you may be expected to select instruments, arrange instruments, and/or perform some other task.
  - Acquaint yourself with the physical facility.
  - If the required procedures are not clear to you, ask for clarification.
- Whether you are taking a written or clinical exam, budget your time.
  - Make a quick overview of the number of tasks required in the clinical exam or the number of questions to be answered in a written exam.
  - Think of the pace you will need to allow the appropriate amount of time to complete each section.
  - Remember that some tasks or questions may require more time than others.
- Many test takers find it wise to work all the way through a written exam at a fairly rapid pace by first answering all the questions they "know" or to which they can work out the answer fairly quickly.
  - This method suggests skipping the tough questions the first time through and coming back to them later.
  - It helps you to build on your own success.
  - Success can help to lessen fears or concerns that you may have about the testing situation.
  - Sometimes the reading of a question in the middle or toward the end of an exam may trigger your mind with the answer or provide an important clue to an earlier question.
- Be certain that if you skip a question you take caution in entering the next answer in the appropriate space; double check the question number with the number on the answer sheet or the computer screen.
- Be cautious when reviewing your answer sheet to not make arbitrary changes in your answers.
  - Be certain to review the question thoroughly before making an answer change.
  - Limited research available suggests that "abler" students tend to increase their test scores "a bit" by carefully reviewing items, whereas lower-scoring students do not. Go back over questions primarily to check that you have not made some obvious error in such things as reading or marking.
- When taking a clinical exam, many of the same principles apply.
  - Proceed cautiously and deliberately, making sure that you understand the task being presented.
  - Be certain to review your work to ensure it meets the clinical criteria before indicating you have completed the tasks.

The credentialing exams available for dental assistants have been designed to allow students to demonstrate knowledge and show their proficiency in skills essential to begin work as dental professionals. Think of the credentialing exam in dental assisting as an opportunity to demonstrate professional competency in your chosen field. Preparation for such an exam is preparation for your chosen profession.

Publisher Acknowledgment

The publisher wishes to thank Betty Ladley Finkbeiner for her expertise and leadership in this project. Her work ethic, commitment to dental education, and many insights were an inspiration to us all.

Contents

General Chairside, Radiation Health and Safety, and Infection Control

General Chairside

Directions: Select the response that is the best answer to each of the following questions. Only one response is correct.

1. The position of the body standing erect with the feet together and the arms hanging at the sides with the palms facing forward is referred to as the _____ position.
   a. resting
   b. anatomic
   c. supine
   d. postural

2. In the illustration shown, Dr. Curtis was assisted by Debbie May Ross to complete operative treatment for this patient. What required data are missing from the chart?
   a. file number or "NA" if not used, date of the appointment, dentist's initials
   b. time of the appointment, amount of cavity medication used, dentist's initials
   c. type of dental material, amount of cavity medication used, assistant's initials
   d. file number or "NA" if not used, assistant's initials

PROGRESS NOTES ▮▮▮▮▮▮▮▮▮▮▮▮▮▮▮▮

Name _____*Whitworth, Kimberly*_____ Birth date *10/27/69* File # _____ Page ___*1*___

11/19/00   19MD   2C Carbo., Life, A   JWC

---

3. The examination technique in which the examiner uses his or her fingers to feel for size, texture, and consistency of hard and soft tissue is called:
   a. determination
   b. palpation
   c. inspection
   d. assessment

4. Which type of consent is given when a patient enters a dentist's office?
   a. informed consent
   b. implied consent
   c. implied consent for minors
   d. informed refusal

5. Consent is:
   a. an involuntary act of submission to dental procedures
   b. a voluntary acceptance of what is planned or done by another person
   c. only necessary for surgical procedures involving general anesthesia
   d. only legal if the patient is older than 21 years of age

6. A patient's chart that denotes a congenital absence of some or all of the teeth would indicate:
   a. micrognathia
   b. ankylosis
   c. macrognathia
   d. anodontia

7. The tooth-numbering system that begins with the maxillary right third molar as tooth #1 and ends with the mandibular right third molar as tooth #32 is the _____ system.
   a. Universal
   b. Palmer Notation
   c. Fédération Dentaire Internationale
   d. Global Numbering

8. An abbreviation used in the progress notes or chart to indicate a mesioocclusobuccal restoration is:
   a. BuOcM
   b. BOM
   c. MOD
   d. MOB

9. A developmental abnormality characterized by the complete bonding of two adjacent teeth caused by irregular growth is:
   a. germination
   b. fusion
   c. ankylosis
   d. concrescence

10. A(n) _____ tooth is any tooth that is prevented from reaching its normal position in the mouth by tissue, bone, or another tooth.
    a. avulsed
    b. impacted
    c. ankylosed
    d. fused

11. An oral habit consisting of involuntary gnashing, grinding, and clenching of the teeth is:
    a. erosion
    b. bruxism
    c. attrition
    d. abrasion

12. A horizontal or transverse plane divides the body into:
    a. superior and inferior portions
    b. dorsal and ventral portions
    c. anterior and posterior portions
    d. medial and lateral portions

13. The cells associated with bone formation are known as:
    a. osteoclasts
    b. cancellous cells
    c. cortical cells
    d. osteoblasts

14. The air/water syringe should be flushed for _____ at the beginning and end of each day.
   a. 30 seconds
   b. 2 minutes
   c. 5 minutes
   d. 30 minutes

15. One of the functions of the paranasal sinuses is to:
   a. aid in digestion
   b. warm inspired air
   c. assist in smelling
   d. absorb bacteria

16. The air/water syringe should be flushed for at least _____ between patients.
   a. 30 seconds
   b. 3 minutes
   c. 5 minutes
   d. 30 minutes

17. Which zone corresponds to the 4 o'clock to 7 o'clock region?
   a. transfer zone
   b. activity zone
   c. assisting zone
   d. static zone

18. A 10-year-old patient would likely have which of the following teeth?
   a. permanent mandibular central and lateral incisors, primary second molars, permanent mandibular canines, and permanent first molars
   b. permanent mandibular central and lateral incisors, permanent first and second premolars, primary second molars, and permanent first molars
   c. primary mandibular central and lateral incisors, primary second molars, permanent canines, and permanent first molars
   d. permanent mandibular canines, primary central and lateral incisors, primary second molars, and permanent first molars

19. What is the average range of the body's oral resting temperature?
   a. 93.5° F to 99.5° F
   b. 95° F to 99.5° F
   c. 96.5° F to 100° F
   d. 97.6° F to 99° F

20. In dentistry the acronym HVE represents:
   a. high-volume evacuation
   b. high-velocity emigration
   c. high-velocity evacuation
   d. high-volume emigration

21. The primary step in preventing a medical emergency is to be certain the patient has _____ before treatment is begun.
   a. eaten
   b. taken all assigned medications
   c. completed and updated his or her medical history
   d. signed a consent form

22. What are the symptoms a patient would display when experiencing a cerebrovascular accident?
    a. paralysis, speech problems, and vision problems
    b. hunger, sweating, and mood change
    c. itching, erythema, and hives
    d. coughing, wheezing, and increased pulse rate

23. The most current adult basic life support protocol (CAB) is an acronym for:
    a. compressions, airway, breathing
    b. circulation, assess, breathing
    c. compressions, assess, breathing
    d. call, assess, breathing

24. The most frequently used substance in a medical emergency is:
    a. glucose
    b. oxygen
    c. epinephrine
    d. ammonia inhalant

25. The leading cause of heart attack is:
    a. rheumatic fever
    b. valvular heart disease
    c. infective endocarditis
    d. coronary artery disease

26. Which of the following is precipitated by stress and anxiety; may manifest in rapid, shallow breathing, lightheadedness, a rapid heartbeat, and a panic-stricken appearance; and is treated by having the patient breathe into a paper bag or cupped hands?
    a. asthma attack
    b. hyperventilation
    c. allergic reaction
    d. angina

27. While you are providing dental treatment for a patient in her third trimester of pregnancy, the patient suddenly feels dizzy and short of breath. How should the patient be repositioned in the dental chair?
    a. supine
    b. tilted to the left side
    c. subsupine
    d. parallel to the floor

28. To ensure that a medical emergency is observed immediately, it is important for the dental assistant to:
    a. check the patient's pulse periodically during treatment
    b. check the patient's blood pressure periodically during treatment
    c. be alert to continuously observe the patient to note any potential problems
    d. ask the patient periodically how he or she feels

29. What are the symptoms a patient would display when experiencing hypoglycemia?
    a. paralysis, speech problems, and vision problems
    b. hunger, sweating, and mood change
    c. itching, erythema, and hives
    d. coughing, wheezing, and increased pulse rate

30. In relation to ergonomics in a dental business office, there are how many classifications of motion?
    a. four
    b. five
    c. three
    d. two

31. The distance between the operator's face and the patient's oral cavity should be approximately _____ inches.
    a. 6
    b. 10
    c. 16
    d. 24

32. While positioned in the dental assisting stool, the dental assistant should rest his or her feet:
    a. on the floor
    b. on the tubular bar around the base of the stool
    c. on the legs of the dental stool
    d. with one foot on the floor and one foot on the stool leg

33. Which of the following medical conditions is considered a contraindication for nitrous oxide analgesia?
    a. severe emotional disturbances
    b. high blood pressure
    c. epilepsy
    d. diabetes

34. Motion economy is the concept that encourages the dental health care worker to:
    a. increase the number and length of motions at chairside
    b. decrease the number and length of motions at chairside
    c. use quick motions to save energy
    d. use slow, deliberate motions that exercise the arm to reduce stress

35. Which of the following instruments would be found on a prophylaxis tray setup?
    a. spoon excavator
    b. burnisher
    c. scaler
    d. pocket marker

36. The lowest level of Maslow's hierarchy of needs is:
    a. physiologic
    b. security
    c. social
    d. self-actualization

37. Which of the following should be done if the patient has thick, heavy saliva that adheres to the prophylaxis cup during the polishing procedure?
    a. place a saliva ejector in the mouth instead of using the HVE tip
    b. keep the HVE tip as close as possible to the polishing cup
    c. do not polish the teeth
    d. have the patient rinse out in the sink after all the polishing is done

38. Plaster of Paris and dental stone are examples of:
   a. impression materials
   b. intermediary materials
   c. gypsum products
   d. impression trays

39. The portion of a bridge that replaces the missing tooth is called a(n):
   a. denture
   b. abutment
   c. pontic
   d. root

40. Which of the following instruments would be used to measure the depth of the gingival sulcus?
   a. periodontal probe
   b. cowhorn explorer
   c. right angle explorer
   d. shepherd's hook

41. Which of the following instruments is used to scale an area specific deep periodontal pocket?
   a. Gracey curette
   b. sickle scaler
   c. spoon excavator
   d. hoe scaler

42. The HVE system is used:
   a. to remove liquids slowly
   b. to remove large volumes of fluid and debris from the mouth
   c. primarily during surgical procedures
   d. most commonly during a prophylaxis

43. Which of the following instruments can be used to invert the rubber dam?
   a. explorer
   b. spoon excavator
   c. svedopter
   d. floss

44. If treatment is to be performed on tooth #13, the clamp is placed on which tooth?
   a. #14 and #14 through #11 are isolated.
   b. #15 and #15 through #12 are isolated.
   c. #13 and #14 through #11 are isolated.
   d. #12 and #12 through #15 are isolated.

45. You are assisting a right-handed operator in a procedure performed on the patient's left side. The HVE tip and A/W syringe are being used. The operator signals for a transfer. You must:
   a. return the A/W to the dental unit, hold onto the HVE, and pick up the new instrument to be transferred
   b. transfer the A/W syringe to the right hand, retain the HVE tip in the right hand, and pick up the new instrument to be transferred
   c. lay both the HVE and A/W syringe across your lap and pick up the new instrument to be transferred
   d. give a signal to the dentist or operator that you are unable to make the transfer at this time

46. Which of the following is the correct statement regarding the seating position of the operator?
    a. The operator's thighs are parallel to the floor.
    b. The operator is seated as far forward on the stool as possible.
    c. The operator is always seated at the 12 o'clock position.
    d. The operator's feet rest on the stool legs.

47. When placing the amalgam into the preparation for a 31DO restoration, the first increment should be placed into the:
    a. distoocclusal region
    b. proximal box
    c. mesioocclusal region
    d. midocclusal region

48. Which of the following instruments would be used to grasp tissue or bone fragments during a surgical procedure?
    a. hemostat
    b. locking endodontic pliers
    c. periosteal elevator
    d. rongeur forceps

49. Which of the following is the common choice in providing for retention in a cavity preparation?
    a. no. 34 high speed
    b. no. 57 low speed
    c. no. 2, 3, or 6 low speed
    d. no. ½ on low or high speed

50. What type of matrix is used for an anterior esthetic restoration?
    a. celluloid strip
    b. straight metal matrix
    c. contoured metal matrix
    d. finishing strip

51. When placing a composite restoration on the buccal cervical of tooth #30, which is the choice of matrix?
    a. universal circumferential metal matrix
    b. class V composite matrix
    c. celluloid strip
    d. celluloid crown

52. The most common form of anesthesia used in operative dentistry is:
    a. local
    b. conscious sedation
    c. inhalation
    d. general

53. For dental professionals, the safest allowable amount of N_2O is _____ parts per million.
    a. 50
    b. 75
    c. 100
    d. 1000

54. Which of the following medical conditions is a contraindication to using a vasoconstrictor in the local anesthesia during operative treatment?
    a. diabetes
    b. recent heart attack
    c. pregnancy
    d. epilepsy

55. _____ is frequently used on the mandibular teeth and is injected near a major nerve that anesthetizes the entire area served by that nerve branch.
    a. Block anesthesia
    b. Infiltration anesthesia
    c. Innervation anesthesia
    d. Induction anesthesia

56. Nitrous oxide oxygen administration always begins and ends with:
    a. the patient deep breathing
    b. the patient breathing 100% oxygen
    c. taking the patient's blood pressure and temperature
    d. providing a glass of water or other cold beverage

57. When there is not enough teeth structure to hold a prosthetic crown, a _____ is used to aid in retention.
    a. matrix band
    b. core buildup
    c. celluloid strip
    d. retention pin

58. The tray setup in the photograph is used to:
    a. place separators
    b. fit and cement orthodontic bands
    c. directly bond orthodontic bands
    d. place and remove ligature ties

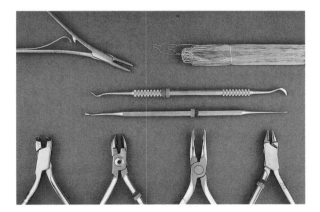

59. To control swelling after a surgical procedure, the patient should be instructed to:
    a. place a cold pack in a cycle of 20 minutes on and 20 minutes off for the first 24 hours
    b. place a cold pack in a cycle of 60 minutes on and 60 minutes off for the first 12 hours
    c. place a cold pack in a cycle of 20 minutes on and 20 minutes off for the first 12 hours and then apply heat in the same form for the next 12 hours
    d. place a heat pack in a cycle of 20 minutes on and 20 minutes off for the first 24 hours

60. The painful condition that can result from the premature loss of a blood clot after a tooth extraction is known as:
a. periodontitis
b. alveolitis
c. hemostasis
d. gingivitis

61. It may take _____ to complete a dental implant procedure.
a. 1 month
b. 6 to 8 weeks
c. 3 to 9 months
d. 1 year

62. A metal frame that is placed under the periosteum and on top of the bone is called a(n):
a. endosteal implant
b. subperiosteal implant
c. transosteal implant
d. triseptal implant

63. The natural rubber material used to obturate the pulp canal after treatment is completed is called:
a. silver point
b. gutta-percha
c. glass ionomer
d. endodontic filler

64. In this photograph, which instrument is a barbed broach?

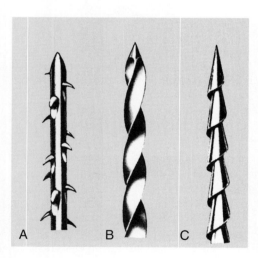

65. A common solution used for irrigation during the debridement procedure in endodontic treatment is:
a. sodium chloride
b. sterile saline solution
c. sodium hypochlorite
d. sterile water

66. The incisional periodontal surgical procedure that does not remove tissues but pushes away the underlying tooth roots and alveolar bone is known as:
    a. gingivectomy
    b. gingivoplasty
    c. flap surgery
    d. apicoectomy

67. According to recent studies, periodontal disease is associated with an increased risk of developing which of the following conditions?
    a. epilepsy
    b. Sjögren syndrome
    c. cardiovascular disease
    d. cleft palate

68. The _____ is an instrument that resembles a large spoon and is used to debride the interior of the socket to remove diseased tissue and abscesses.
    a. root tip elevator
    b. rongeur
    c. surgical curette
    d. hemostat

69. From the instruments shown here, select the curette.

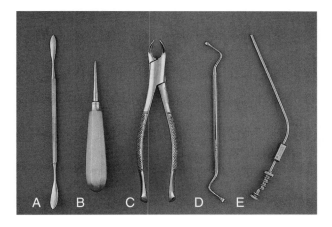

70. Coronal polishing is a technique used to remove_____ from tooth surfaces.
    a. supragingival calculus
    b. intrinsic stain
    c. plaque
    d. cement

71. What terms are used to classify stain by location?
    a. exogenous and endogenous
    b. extrinsic and intrinsic
    c. endogenous and intrinsic
    d. exogenous and extrinsic

72. The purpose of using disclosing solution is to _____
    a. identify calculus
    b. visualize plaque
    c. desensitize tooth structure
    d. destroy bacteria

73. The first step in placing dental sealants is to _____ the surface.
    a. etch
    b. isolate
    c. clean
    d. prime

74. Enamel that has been etched has the appearance of being:
    a. chalky
    b. shiny
    c. wet
    d. slightly brown

75. Which of the following medical emergencies would be treated with a bronchodilator?
    a. epileptic seizure
    b. cerebrovascular accident
    c. asthma attack
    d. hypoglycemic incident

76. The isolation of multiple anterior teeth requires the dental dam be placed _____.
    a. only on the one tooth being restored
    b. on the tooth being restored and on one tooth distal on each side
    c. from premolar to premolar
    d. from first molar to first molar

77. During a dental procedure, the dental assistant's stool is _____ the operator's stool.
    a. lower than
    b. higher than
    c. same height as
    d. even with

78. Gingival retraction cord is placed _____ the crown preparation is completed and is removed _____ the final impression is taken.
    a. after, after
    b. before, before
    c. before, after
    d. after, before

79. A _____ is an orthodontic _____ that is a custom appliance made of rubber or pliable acrylic that fits over the patient's dentition after orthodontic treatment.
    a. Harding retainer, arch wire
    b. Hawley retainer, fixed appliance
    c. headgear, positioner
    d. Hawley retainer, positioner

80. This tray setup is for:
   a. band removal
   b. placing and removing elastomeric ties
   c. placing separators
   d. placing arch wires

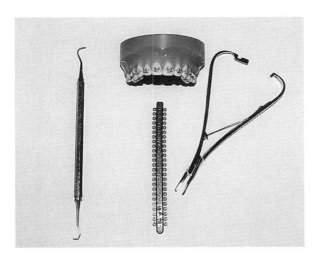

81. Instrument "A" in the photograph is used to:
   a. insert the orthodontic band
   b. force the band down onto the middle third of the tooth
   c. aid in forcing the cement out of the band
   d. open the buccal tube

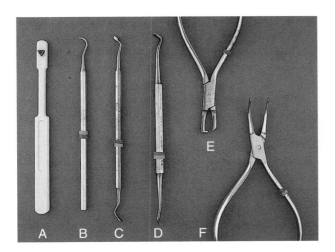

82. A(n) _____ is used to provide interproximal space for inserting an orthodontic band.
   a. arch wire
   b. bracket
   c. separator
   d. band

83. Which of the following is a rotary device used with discs or wheels?
   a. bur
   b. ultrasonic
   c. prophy angle
   d. mandrel

84. When instructing a patient about treatment for angular cheilitis, where would the dental assistant tell the patient to place the topical antibiotic?
   a. oral mucosa
   b. floor of mouth
   c. commissure of the lips
   d. lateral borders of tongue

85. When describing a superficial infection caused by a yeast-like fungus to a patient, what would you call this condition?
   a. leukoplakia
   b. lichen planus
   c. candidiasis
   d. aphthous ulcer

86. Which instrument would be used to remove the right mandibular first molar?

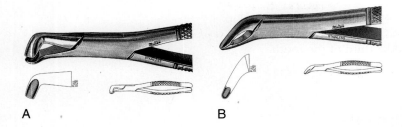

A   B

87. Which instrument would be used to remove the right maxillary second molar?

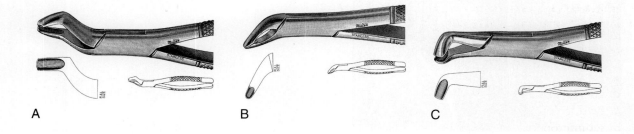

A   B   C

88. Which of the following instruments would be used to remove a metal matrix band after carving an amalgam restoration?
   a. shepherd's hook explorer
   b. rubber dam forceps
   c. acorn burnisher
   d. cotton forceps

89. When a tooth is avulsed, it has:
   a. been fractured
   b. come out
   c. been pushed back into the socket
   d. become loose

90. An automated external defibrillator (AED) is used for what medical emergency?
   a. sudden cardiac arrest
   b. respiratory distress
   c. epileptic seizure
   d. diabetic coma

91. One of the characteristics that allows gold to be one of the most compatible restorative materials in the oral environment is the ability to:
   a. resist tarnishing
   b. be triturated
   c. become corrosive
   d. produce allergens

92. A dental restorative material that is applied to a tooth or teeth while the material is pliable and can be adapted, carved, and finished is classified as:
   a. direct restorations
   b. indirect restorations
   c. crowns, bridges, or onlays
   d. implants

93. Which of these would have the least dimensional stability?
   a. silicone
   b. polysiloxane
   c. alginate hydrocolloid
   d. agar hydrocolloid

94. The conventional or traditional composites, which contain the largest filler particles and provide the greatest strength, are known as:
   a. microfilled composites
   b. hybrid composites
   c. midfilled composites
   d. macrofilled composites

95. If a light–bodied impression catalyst is mixed with a heavy-bodied impression base, the resultant mix might:
   a. be discolored
   b. set improperly
   c. polymerize immediately
   d. not mix

96. Addition of cold water to an alginate mix will cause the setting time to be:
   a. increased
   b. shortened
   c. reduced
   d. unaffected

97. Select two terms that describe the purpose and consistency of a dental cement used for the final seating of a porcelain fused-to-metal crown.
   a. base and secondary consistency
   b. cementation and secondary consistency
   c. base and primary consistency
   d. cementation and primary consistency

98. Which of the following is a noble metal?
   a. tin
   b. iron
   c. zinc
   d. palladium

99. The purpose of calcium hydroxide in a cavity preparation is to:
   a. release fluoride to prevent decay
   b. help the formation of reparative dentin
   c. create a bond to the restorative material
   d. cover the smear layer

100. The advantage of using a glass ionomer as a restorative material is that it:
   a. helps the formation of reparative dentin
   b. releases fluoride after its final setting
   c. can be easily matched to any tooth color
   d. relieves toothaches because it contains oil of clove

101. A custom tray is constructed to fit the mouth of a specific patient and is used to _____, _____, and _____.
   a. save money, reduce chair time, reduce patient discomfort
   b. adapt to the patient's mouth, fit around any anomalies, reduce the amount of impression material needed
   c. adapt to the patient's mouth, aid the laboratory technician, provide for a better restoration
   d. reduce patient cost, reduce chair time, reduce patient discomfort

102. Which form of gypsum product is commonly used for making diagnostic models?
   a. plaster
   b. dental stone
   c. high-strength stone
   d. impression plaster

103. When taking impressions, the next step after seating the patient and placing the patient napkin is to:
   a. assemble the materials needed
   b. mix the impression material
   c. explain the procedure to the patient
   d. record treatment on the chart

104. Which of the following instruments is used to cut soft tissue during a tooth extraction?
   a. surgical curette
   b. tissue retractor
   c. scalpel
   d. hemostat

105. Vital information on a registration form includes the _____ of the person responsible for the account.
    a. name, address, and phone number
    b. military service and type of discharge
    c. race, citizenship, and national origin
    d. height, weight, and picture

106. Financial arrangements for dental treatment should be made:
    a. at the reception desk by the dental assistant
    b. only if the patient has dental insurance
    c. before treatment is started
    d. by the dental insurance company

107. _____ is the amount the dental assistant takes home after all deductions are made.
    a. Gross pay
    b. Net pay
    c. Withholding
    d. FICA

108. _____ is another name for the Social Security funds deducted from an employee's pay.
    a. Withholding
    b. FICA
    c. Federal tax
    d. Gross wage

109. Which of these is an expendable item used in the dental office?
    a. hemostat
    b. instrument cassette
    c. latex gloves
    d. computer software

110. Which is a capital item in a dental office?
    a. hemostat
    b. cotton rolls
    c. x-ray unit
    d. computer software

111. Oxygen should be stored:
    a. horizontally in a cool place
    b. vertically and secured
    c. horizontally in a warm place
    d. outside the office

112. An office system that tracks patients' follow-up visits for an oral prophylaxis is a(n):
    a. screening system
    b. on-call record
    c. recall system
    d. tickler file

113. Which of the following statements should be reworded on a patient's record to avoid litigation?
    a. The patient experienced difficulty in holding the impression in the mouth.
    b. The patient was not accustomed to the new laser system used for the procedure.
    c. This patient was a real problem and disrupted our entire day.
    d. The patient apologized for being unable to hold the impression long enough.

114. What are the consequences of using a nickname or an incorrect name when filing an insurance claim form?
    a. No payment will ever be made.
    b. Processing of the form will be delayed.
    c. There are no consequences.
    d. There will be an underpayment.

115. Which of the following instruments is used to remove a tooth in one piece with the crown and root intact?
    a. periosteal elevator
    b. forceps
    c. surgical curette
    d. rongeur

116. Which of the following burs is used to reduce the subgingival margin of a tooth during crown preparation?
    a. flame diamond
    b. finishing
    c. round
    d. inverted cone

117. The leading cause of tooth loss in adults is:
    a. dental caries
    b. aging
    c. periodontal disease
    d. lack of home care

118. The first step in patient education is to:
    a. instruct the patient how to remove plaque
    b. select home care aids
    c. listen carefully to the patient
    d. reinforce home care

119. What would be a good source of protein for a person who eats a vegan diet?
    a. egg
    b. steak
    c. legumes
    d. carrots

120. Which of the following topical anesthetics is the most widely used topical agent in dentistry?
    a. articaine
    b. benzocaine
    c. bupivacaine
    d. levobupivacaine

Radiation Health and Safety

Directions: Select the response that best answers each of the following questions. Only one response is correct.

1. Which of the following statements relates to working with a special needs patient?
   a. Offering assistance is demeaning to special needs patients.
   b. Speaking directly to a patient with a disability is appropriate.
   c. Address questions to the caregiver rather than the patient with a disability.
   d. Intraoral radiographs are recommended for patients with developmental disabilities.

2. Which of the following is a result of incorrect position-indicating device (PID) positioning?
   a. Herringbone
   b. Missing proximal surface
   c. Overlap
   d. Double exposure

3. What is the remedy to prevent overlapped contact areas on a radiographic image?
   a. Use a faster film speed.
   b. Increase the vertical angulation.
   c. Decrease the vertical angulation.
   d. Adjust the horizontal angulation.

4. What technique error will always be present on an occlusal radiograph using size 4 film?
   a. Cone-cut
   b. Elongation
   c. Foreshortening
   d. Overlapped contact areas

5. What is the function of intensifying screens used in extraoral radiography?
   a. To increase the sharpness of the image
   b. To decrease the magnification of the image
   c. To help the patient remain still during the exposure
   d. To decrease the exposure to radiation for the patient

6. What is the term used to describe the area of ideal focus on a panoramic machine?
   a. Cephalostat
   b. Focal trough
   c. Frankfort plane
   d. Midsagittal plane

7. Which statement is true regarding the production of ghost images?
   a. It appears on the opposite side of the real object.
   b. It obscures diagnostic information on the panoramic image.
   c. It may be seen if the patient's earrings are not removed before exposure.
   d. All of the above are true regarding ghost images.

8. What type of radiograph should be prescribed when interproximal dental caries are suspected?
 a. Occlusal
 b. Bite-wing
 c. Periapical
 d. Panoramic

9. What type of image shows the entire tooth, including the apex and surrounding structures?
 a. Skull
 b. Occlusal
 c. Bite-wing
 d. Periapical

10. What is the proper technique to expose a bite-wing radiograph on a patient with mandibular tori?
 a. The receptor is placed on the tori.
 b. The receptor is placed on the tongue.
 c. The receptor is placed between the tori and the tongue.
 d. Intraoral placement is not recommended on patients with mandibular tori.

11. A size 1 intraoral receptor used on an adult patient would most likely image what area?
 a. Maxillary molars
 b. Maxillary incisors
 c. Maxillary premolars
 d. Mandibular premolars

12. The following diagram depicts what type of extraoral radiographic technique?
 a. Cephalometric
 b. Posteroanterior
 c. Transorbital
 d. Submentovertex

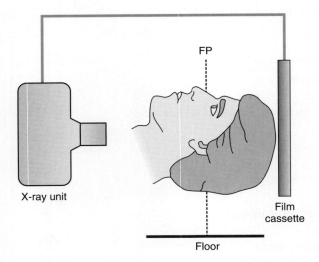

13. What effect will occur by increasing the kilovoltage peak setting on the exposure control panel?
 a. It increases the number of x-rays produced.
 b. It increases the penetrating power of the x-ray beam.
 c. It increases the speed of the photons from anode to cathode.
 d. It decreases the speed of the photons from cathode to anode.

14. Why is insulating oil added to the metal housing of the x-ray tubehead?
   a. To coat the x-ray tube
   b. To absorb excess heat production
   c. To filter the low energy wavelengths
   d. To alter the voltage of incoming electricity

15. The sharpness of a radiographic image is influenced by all of the following factors EXCEPT one. Which one is the EXCEPTION?
   a. Focal spot size
   b. Film composition
   c. Patient movement
   d. Target-to-film distance

16. What type of radiograph is preferred to evaluate for a mandibular jaw fracture?
   a. Occlusal
   b. Bite-wing
   c. Periapical
   d. Panoramic

17. In which situation would extraoral radiography NOT be used?
   a. To evaluate growth and development
   b. To evaluate impacted teeth
   c. To diagnose dental caries
   d. To evaluate the extent of large lesions

18. When exposing a molar bite-wing, the following conditions should exist EXCEPT:
   a. the occlusal plane should be parallel to the floor.
   b. a bite-wing tab should be placed on the receptor.
   c. the receptor should be centered on the first molar.
   d. the central beam should be directed through the contact areas of the molars.

19. An anterior periapical receptor is oriented _____, and a posterior periapical receptor is oriented _____:
   a. vertically; horizontally
   b. horizontally; vertically
   c. vertically; vertically
   d. horizontally; horizontally

20. Which rule governs the orientation of structures portrayed in two radiographs exposed at different angulations?
   a. ALARA
   b. Buccal object rule
   c. SLOB
   d. Right angle rule

21. What piece of equipment is required to hold the receptor parallel to the long axis of the tooth in the paralleling technique?
   a. Bite-wing tab
   b. Receptor holder
   c. Cotton roll
   d. Patient finger

22. All of the following statements regarding duplicating film are true except one. What is the EXCEPTION?
  a. Duplicating film is sensitive to light.
  b. Duplicating film is a double-emulsion film.
  c. The duplicating process is performed in the darkroom.
  d. A duplicating machine is a necessary piece of equipment.

23. Which of the following is NOT considered a critical organ with regards to dental radiography?
  a. Skin
  b. Lens of the eye
  c. Pituitary gland
  d. Bone marrow

24. When is a lead apron used?
  a. When performing a panoramic image
  b. When producing a full mouth series
  c. When performing a periapical exam
  d. All of the above

25. A 5-year-old child fell while playing and needs a periapical radiograph of the anterior region of her maxilla. The child is very upset and uncooperative in the chair. Which of the following is the appropriate action?
  a. Educate the patient to understand why she needs to stay still.
  b. Ask the mother to wait in the reception area.
  c. Have another assistant push the button while you hold the receptor in the patient's mouth.
  d. Have the child hold the x-ray in her mouth.
  e. Have the child sit in the father's lap and drape both in the lead apron.

26. What does ALARA stand for?
  a. As little amount of radiation attainable
  b. As low as reasonably achievable
  c. As low as reasonably allowable
  d. None of the above

27. Which of the following applies to producing radiographs on pregnant patients?
  a. Radiographs should be taken only during the third trimester.
  b. Radiographs should never be taken on a pregnant patient.
  c. Guidelines are designed to protect the patient; no alterations need to be applied.
  d. Radiographs should only be taken during the first trimester.

28. What is the maximum permissible dose a nonoccupationally exposed individual is allowed to accumulate in a year?
  a. 5.0 rem
  b. 0.1 rem
  c. 1.0 rem
  d. 0.01 rem

29. What is the single best way to protect a patient from unnecessary radiation exposure?
  a. Correct collimation
  b. Fast film technique
  c. Use of lead apron
  d. Correct exposure settings

30. Which collimator and PID reduce the amount of exposure a patient receives?
   a. Round and 8 inch
   b. Rectangular and 8 inch
   c. Round and 16 inch
   d. Rectangular and 16 inch

31. Equipment filtration is comprised of which of the following?
   1. Inherent filtration
   2. Added filtration
   3. Total filtration
   a. 1, 2, 3
   b. 2, 3
   c. 1, 3
   d. 1, 2

32. What is the role of a collimator?
   a. Restricting beam size
   b. Confining the beam
   c. Restricting the size and shape of the beam
   d. Reducing short wavelengths

33. How are film-holding devices used to protect the patient from exposure?
   a. They stabilize the film position in the mouth and reduce the chance for movement.
   b. XCPs are the easiest system to use.
   c. They are easier for the patient to bite.
   d. They are more comfortable for the patient thus resulting in less retakes.

34. Which of the following is true about the exposure of radiation on the body?
   a. Brings about changes to body chemicals, tissues, organs, and cells
   b. Brings about changes to tissues, organs, and cells
   c. Brings about changes to body chemicals, tissues, and organs
   d. None of the above

35. Which source produces the most annual radiation exposure to persons in the United States?
   a. Radon
   b. Cosmic
   c. Terrestrial
   d. Medical or dental

36. The following diagram depicts the correct positioning of the PID (position-indicating device) _____.

    a. for bisecting angle

    b. in the horizontal plane

    c. to prevent elongation

    d. to prevent foreshortening

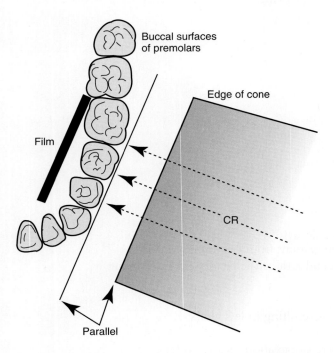

37. What is the size of the x-ray beam produced by a circular collimator as it reaches the patient's face?

    a. 1.75 inches

    b. 2.50 inches

    c. 2.75 inches

    d. 3.25 inches

38. Which PID would provide the most protection against radiation exposure for the patient?

    a. Plastic, round

    b. Plastic, conical

    c. Lead-lined, round

    d. Lead-lined, rectangular

39. What is the purpose of including aluminum filtration inside the dental tubehead?

    a. To direct the x-ray beam

    b. To restrict the size and shape of the x-ray beam

    c. To remove the low energy x-rays from the beam

    d. To protect the reproductive tissues from scatter radiation

40. Which of the following would be considered a short-term effect of radiation exposure?

    a. Nausea

    b. Genetic defects

    c. Cancer induction

    d. Birth abnormalities

41. What is the term to describe the time between radiation exposure and the appearance of the first clinical signs?
    a. Latent period
    b. Period of injury
    c. Recovery period
    d. Cumulative exposures

42. Which cell would be considered radio-resistant?
    a. Skin
    b. Muscle
    c. Oral mucosa
    d. Reproductive cells

43. When the dental operator is producing a radiographic image on a patient, it is recommended that he or she stand at least how far away from the primary beam?
    a. 5 feet
    b. 6 inches
    c. 2 feet
    d. 6 feet

44. What is the maximum permissible dose an occupationally exposed radiographer is allowed to accumulate in a year?
    a. 5.0 rem
    b. 0.01 rem
    c. 1.0 rem
    d. 3.0 rem

45. What can a radiographer wear to measure the daily amount of radiation exposure?
    a. Rad badge
    b. DEP monitoring badge
    c. Dosimeter badge
    d. None of the above

46. Of the three forms of radiation, which is most detrimental to the patient and operator?
    a. Primary, secondary, and scatter radiation
    b. Primary and secondary radiation
    c. Secondary radiation
    d. Scatter radiation

47. Why is it important for a radiographer to understand ionizing radiation?
    a. Ionizing radiation causes harmful effects to humans.
    b. Ionizing radiation causes damage to the cellular metabolism.
    c. All of the above.
    d. None of the above.

48. What is the best way for the dental operator to prevent exposure to x-radiation?
    a. Avoid the primary beam.
    b. Do not hold the receptor in place for the patient.
    c. Stand around the corner from the radiology cubicle.
    d. Stand at least 3 feet away from the x-ray tubehead.

49. Which of the following statements relates to working with a patient with a physical challenge or one with special needs?
    a. Offering assistance is demeaning to patients with special needs.
    b. Speaking directly to a patient with a disability is appropriate.
    c. Address questions to the caregiver rather than the patient with a disability.
    d. Intraoral radiographs are recommended for patients with developmental disabilities.

50. Which of the following is an advantage of digital radiography?
    a. The diagnostic quality of digital radiography is compromised by the amount of x-radiation required.
    b. Digital radiography eliminates the need for a darkroom and processing procedures.
    c. Digital radiography eliminates the potential for cone cutting and image cutoff.
    d. The typical sensor in digital radiography is less sensitive to x-rays than conventional film.

51. What technique should the dental assistant use on a patient with a gag reflex?
    a. Tell the patient to hold his or her breath.
    b. Try to reduce tactile stimuli.
    c. Use the term "gagging" when talking with the patient.
    d. Do not try to distract the patient.

52. What is the traditional statute of limitations for adult radiographs?
    a. 5 years
    b. 7 years
    c. 10 years
    d. 12 years

53. Which device is used to restrict the size and shape of the x-ray beam and to reduce patient exposure?
    a. Inherent filtration
    b. Added filtration
    c. Collimation
    d. PID

54. What is the purpose of a dosimeter?
    a. To protect the patient from stray radiation
    b. To measure individual exposures to radiation
    c. To measure cumulative exposure to radiation
    d. To protect pregnant women from exposure to radiation

55. Commercially available barrier envelopes _____.
    a. minimize contamination before exposure of the film
    b. minimize contamination after exposure of the film
    c. are made of a material that blocks the passage of photons
    d. are made of a material that blocks the passage of electrons

56. Which type of PID would be most effective in reducing patient exposure?
    a. Conical
    b. 16-inch round PID
    c. 8-inch rectangular PID
    d. 16-inch rectangular PID

57. The time interval between radiographic examinations for children should be _____.
    a. every 6 months
    b. every 12 months
    c. biannually
    d. based on the individual needs of the child

58. Which of the following is the greatest source of cross-contamination in dental radiology?
   a. The operator's hands
   b. The film packet
   c. The lead apron
   d. The beam alignment device

59. Which of the following is a result of improper storage of x-ray film?
   a. Grayish film
   b. Clear film
   c. Black film
   d. White film

60. Which of the following is recommended by the CDC?
   a. Immersion of film packets in disinfecting solutions
   b. Disinfecting with at least a low-level EPA registered disinfectant
   c. Cold-sterilizing semicritical items
   d. The operator wearing mask and eye protection

61. Which of the following components of the tubehead protects the patient by removing long-wave energy?
   a. Window
   b. Filter
   c. Lead-lined PID
   d. Collimator

62. Which of the following would be helpful to a patient who is uncertain about having dental radiographs taken?
   a. An explanation of the insurance benefits
   b. Prescreening of the patient for a gag reflex
   c. An explanation of the difference between wet and dry processing
   d. Patient education on the value of radiographs

63. One of the greatest services a dental professional can provide for patients is a:_____.
   a. properly taken medical history
   b. comprehensive dental health education
   c. thoroughly documented oral examination
   d. high-quality series of dental radiographs

64. Packaged dental radiography film is affected by all except:_____.
   a. heat
   b. humidity
   c. radiation
   d. ultraviolet light

65. Which of the following describes the frequency with which processing solutions must be changed?
   a. Every 3-4 weeks
   b. Every 5-6 weeks
   c. Every 7-8 weeks
   d. As films begin to appear light

66. A yellow-brown color on a developed film would indicate which of the following?
    a. Exhausted developer
    b. Exhausted fixer
    c. Dirty processing tank
    d. Water temperature that is too warm

67. The optimal storage temperature for dental film is: _____.
    a. 45-50 degrees F
    b. 50-70 degrees F
    c. 73-79 degrees F
    d. 80-85 degrees F

68. When stocking dental radiographic film, it is best to apply which of the following rules of thumb?
    a. Last-in, first-out
    b. First-in, last-out
    c. First-in, first-out
    d. Use all out-of-date film first

69. When intensifying screens are not in perfect contact with the screen film, which of the following will result?
    a. The screen may be damaged.
    b. The film may be damaged.
    c. A loss of image sharpness will occur.
    d. The film will be very dark.

70. Sodium sulfite in the developer solution is responsible for_____.
    a. converting exposed silver halide crystals to black metallic silver
    b. preventing rapid oxidation of the developing agent
    c. activating the developer agents
    d. softening the gelatin of the film emulsion

71. Creating an identical copy of a set of radiographs is called _____.
    a. film duplication
    b. twinning
    c. copying
    d. mirroring

72. Uses of duplicate films include all EXCEPT _____.
    a. insurance submission
    b. copy for the patient to keep
    c. referral to a specialist
    d. teaching

73. The improper exposure of a dental radiograph may result in which of the following?
    a. Phobia
    b. Malpractice
    c. Standard of care
    d. Insurance fraud

74. Informed consent implies that the patient has received _____.
   a. some disclosure
   b. no disclosure
   c. complete disclosure
   d. enough disclosure

75. The dental record is a legal document.
   a. True
   b. False

76. Which of the following is the final step in film duplication?
   a. Label the radiographic mount.
   b. Arrange the radiographs on the light source.
   c. Place the duplicating film on the arranged radiographs.
   d. Secure the lid and set the timer.

77. The longer duplicating film is exposed to light, _____.
   a. the darker it appears
   b. the more opaque it appears
   c. the lighter it appears
   d. the more translucent it appears

78. A blurred image on a duplication film is likely caused by which of the following?
   a. Slippage
   b. Poor contact between the source image and the duplicating film
   c. Incorrect time
   d. Bad duplication film quality

79. Used developer solution must be disposed of in which of the following ways?
   a. In a leak-proof biohazard bag
   b. Flushed down the sanitary drain sewer
   c. Placed in the septic system
   d. Placed in a special container to be picked up by a special service

80. Which of the following infection control protocols applies to radiography procedures?
   a. Standard precautions need to be followed.
   b. A face mask does not need to be worn during procedures.
   c. Patients should wear protective eyewear.
   d. Utility gloves should be worn during cleanup and disinfection procedures.

81. Dental x-ray equipment is classified as _____.
   a. critical instruments
   b. semicritical instruments
   c. noncritical instruments
   d. semcritical and noncritical instruments

82. Prior to dental film exposure, which of the following must be covered or disinfected?
   a. X-ray machine
   b. Beam alignment device
   c. Towel dispenser
   d. Image receptor

83. Which is a correct statement concerning disinfection procedures for the darkroom?
    a. Countertops and areas touched by gloved hands must be disinfected.
    b. Countertops do not need to be disinfected, as no aerosolization occurs in the process of dental x-ray films.
    c. Countertops need to be covered with a barrier before each clinical use and discarded at the end of the day.
    d. A high-level disinfectant is required to disinfect the area surrounding the processor.

84. EPA-registered chemical germicides labeled as a *tuberculocidal* are classified as _____.
    a. high-level disinfectants
    b. intermediate-level disinfectants
    c. low-level disinfectants

85. Films removed from barrier envelopes are processed with _____.
    a. gloved hands
    b. ungloved hands
    c. powder-free gloves
    d. utility gloves

86. Beam alignment devices must be _____.
    a. sterilized
    b. disinfected
    c. decontaminated
    d. wiped with alcohol between use

87. The three types of hand hygiene advised for radiography procedures include all EXCEPT which of the following?
    a. Routine handwashing
    b. Aseptic hand wash
    c. Antiseptic handwashing
    d. Antiseptic hand rub

88. A needle-stick injury would result in which type of exposure to infectious disease?
    a. Occupational exposure
    b. Parenteral exposure
    c. Critical exposure
    d. Semicritical exposure

89. An instrument used to penetrate soft tissue or bone is considered a _____ instrument.
    a. critical
    b. semicritical
    c. noncritical
    d. semicritical and noncritical

90. Which statement is correct concerning the use of gloves during a radiography procedure?
    a. Gloves must be washed prior to use to remove powder residue.
    b. Gloves must be sterile for all procedures.
    c. New gloves must be worn for each patient.
    d. Gloves must be worn only when contact with saliva is anticipated.

91. Which of the following statements is correct regarding the use of masks and protective eyewear during radiographic procedures?
   a. Face masks are required but protective eyewear is not.
   b. Protective eyewear is required but face masks are not.
   c. Protective eyewear and face masks are optional.
   d. All PPE, including face masks and protective eyewear, must be worn at all times. Standard Precautions apply.

92. At the end of the radiography procedure, the operator should remove the lead apron from the patient with hands that are _____.
   a. gloved
   b. ungloved
   c. gloved with powder-free gloves

93. Dental films contaminated with saliva should be _____.
   a. placed in an envelope bearing the patient's name
   b. placed in a cup bearing the patient's name
   c. wiped free of saliva with an intermediate-level disinfectant
   d. wiped free of saliva with alcohol

94. Infection control procedures in dental radiography can be divided into which segments/categories?
   a. Before exposure, during exposure, after exposure, processing
   b. Before exposure, processing, interpretation
   c. After exposure, processing, mounting, interpretation
   d. Before exposure, processing, mounting, interpretation

95. The protocol that protects patients from cross-contamination in a radiographic procedure is _____.
   a. Standard Precautions
   b. sterilization of critical instruments
   c. disinfection of critical instruments
   d. use of a lead apron

96. Bite guides of the panoramic or cephalometric x-ray machine should be _____.
   a. sterilized
   b. single-use-only
   c. disinfected
   d. A and B
   e. A and C

97. Beam alignment devices can be placed on _____.
   a. disinfected surfaces
   b. uncovered surfaces
   c. covered surfaces
   d. A, B, and C
   e. A and C

98. The operator should clean and disinfect any uncovered areas while wearing _____.
   a. vinyl gloves
   b. latex gloves
   c. utility gloves
   d. powderless gloves

99. To what radiopaque landmark are the arrows pointing?
   a. Mental ridge
   b. Torus mandibularis
   c. Genial tubercles
   d. Mylohyoid ridge

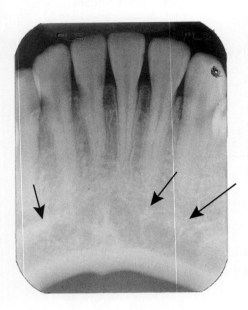

100. This radiograph is an example of which processing error?
   a. Reticulation
   b. Fixer spots
   c. Developer spots
   d. Air bubbles

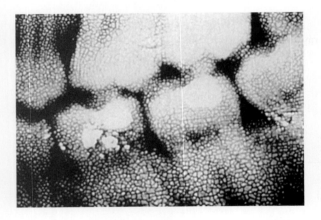

Infection Control

Directions: Select the response that best answers each of the following questions. Only one response is correct.

1. After accepting employment you opt not to receive a hepatitis B vaccination and have signed a waiver to this effect. You have the right to:
   a. change your mind and have the vaccination at your own expense
   b. change your mind and the employer is required to provide the vaccination
   c. demand periodic blood tests to ensure noninvasion of the hepatitis B virus in your body
   d. sue the employer if you contact hepatitis B

2. All dental professionals must use surgical masks and protective eyewear to protect the eyes and face:
   a. only during surgical procedures
   b. whenever the high-speed handpiece is used
   c. whenever spatter and aerosolized sprays of blood and saliva are likely
   d. whenever available

3. All dental assistants involved in direct patient care must undergo routine training in:
   a. infection control, safety issues, and hazard communication
   b. charting, taking patients vital signs, and using the office intercom system
   c. infection control, uniform sizing, and ordering of disposables
   d. hazardous waste management, charting, and application of dental dams

4. When immunity is present at birth, it is referred to as:
   a. acquired immunity
   b. active immunity
   c. artificially acquired immunity
   d. inherited immunity

5. _____ immunity occurs when a vaccination is administered and the body forms antibodies in response to the vaccine.
   a. Active natural
   b. Active artificial
   c. Passive natural
   d. Passive artificial

6. A chronic infection is best exemplified by which of the following?
   a. human immunodeficiency virus
   b. cold sore
   c. common cold
   d. pneumonia

7. Which of the following exemplifies an acute infection?
   a. hepatitis C virus
   b. hepatitis B virus
   c. common cold
   d. pneumonia

8. Microorganisms that produce disease in humans are known as:
   a. nonpathogenic
   b. pathogens
   c. pasteurized
   d. germs

9. Bacteria can be identified by shape. Which of the following is the shape of bacilli?
   a. spherical
   b. rod
   c. spiral
   d. triangular

10. An infection that results from a defective immune system that cannot defend against pathogens normally found in the environment is a(n):
   a. chronic infection
   b. latent infection
   c. acute infection
   d. opportunistic infection

11. Which of the following is an example of parenteral disease transmission in dentistry?
   a. touching or contact with patient's blood or other body fluids
   b. touching or contact with a contaminated surface
   c. contagious droplet infection occurring through mucosal surfaces of the eyes, nose, or mouth
   d. needle stick injury, cuts, abrasions, or any break in the skin

12. The transmission of a disease to a susceptible person by handling contaminated instruments or by touching the face, eyes, or mouth is referred to as:
   a. airborne transmission
   b. direct transmission
   c. indirect transmission
   d. spatter transmission

13. Which of the following would be considered the best method for determining whether there is proper sterilization function of a sterilizer?
   a. a chemically treated tape used on packages that changes color
   b. the time, temperature, and pressure used
   c. a biological spore test through a monitoring system
   d. autoclave bags

14. When a package of hazardous infectious waste is being prepared for disposal, which of the following should be considered?
   a. All infectious waste destined for disposal should be placed in closable, leak-proof containers or bags that are color coded or labeled appropriately.
   b. Infectious waste should be burned in a local incinerator.
   c. Only the clinical assistant should manage the removal of infectious waste.
   d. Only the office manager should manage the removal of infectious waste.

15. Which of the following PPE is removed first after the completion of a clinical procedure?
   a. gloves
   b. protective eyewear
   c. gown
   d. mask

16. Exam gloves used during dental treatment can be made of:
   a. latex
   b. thin plastic
   c. dermal cloth
   d. heavy nitrile

17. Which of the following is considered regulated waste (biohazard)?
   a. spent fixer solution
   b. pathologic waste
   c. paper mixing pad
   d. used barriers

18. Which of the following statements is true as it applies to the use of overgloves?
   a. Overgloves are worn when an assistant has an allergy to latex.
   b. Overgloves are placed before the secondary procedure is performed and are removed before patient treatment is resumed.
   c. Overgloves are made of latex.
   d. Overgloves are acceptable alone as a hand barrier in nonsurgical procedures.

19. During which of the following procedures would you use sterile surgical gloves?
   a. placement of a composite
   b. oral surgery
   c. all bonding procedures
   d. removal of a suture

20. The most common route of disease transmission in the dental office is through:
   a. droplet infection
   b. direct contact with the patient's blood or saliva
   c. indirect contact with surfaces
   d. any dental instruments

21. The strength of an organism in its ability to produce disease is:
   a. virulence
   b. bioburden
   c. pathogens
   d. infectious disease

22. The use of a preprocedural mouth rinse can lower the number of microorganisms that may escape a patient's mouth through which of the following routes?
   a. aerosols
   b. touching the patient napkin
   c. used instrument
   d. indirect contact

23. _____ infection is the mode of disease transmission that involves large-particle droplet spatter. _____ infection involves minute particles that can remain in the air for hours and can be inhaled.
   a. Airborne, Indirect
   b. Airborne, Droplet
   c. Droplet, Aerosol
   d. Airborne, Direct

24. Pathogens that are carried in the blood and body fluids of infected individuals and that can be transmitted to others are referred to as:
    a. bloodborne
    b. parenteral
    c. virulent
    d. acquired

25. Recommendations concerning gloves would fall under which of the following categories of infection control practices that directly relate to dental radiography procedures?
    a. protective attire and barrier techniques
    b. hand washing and care of hands
    c. sterilization or disinfection of instruments
    d. cleaning and disinfection of dental unit and environmental surfaces

26. Protective clothing:
    a. must prevent skin and mucous membrane exposure when contact with blood or other bodily fluids is anticipated
    b. must be worn by clinical and business staff members
    c. should be worn home and laundered daily
    d. must be purchased by the employer

27. When using medical latex or vinyl gloves, _____.
    a. gloves may be rewashed between patients and reused until damaged
    b. nonsterile gloves are recommended for examinations and noninvasive procedures
    c. hands should not be washed before gloving
    d. hands should not be washed between patients

28. _____ is defined as the absence of pathogens, or disease-causing microorganisms.
    a. Antiseptic
    b. Antibiotic
    c. Antiinfective
    d. Asepsis

29. Define antiseptic.
    a. the absence of pathogens or disease-causing microorganisms
    b. a substance that inhibits the growth of bacteria
    c. the use of a chemical or physical procedure to inhibit or destroy pathogens
    d. the act of sterilizing

30. While taking a patient's health history, it is noted that there is a history of tuberculosis and the patient is currently experiencing symptoms of this disease. Which of the following would *not* be appropriate action in the office?
    a. The patient should be referred promptly for medical evaluation of possible infectiousness.
    b. Tell the patient you will not be able to treat him or her anymore.
    c. Defer elective treatment until a physician confirms that the patient does not have infectious tuberculosis.
    d. If urgent dental care must be provided for the patient and it is determined there is infectious tuberculosis, obtain care that can be provided in a tuberculosis isolation center.

31. When can a liquid sterilant or high-level disinfectant achieve sterilization?
   a. only when the solution is used at temperatures above 121° C
   b. when the solution is used only for the longer exposure times
   c. as soon as the minimal exposure time is reached
   d. only when the solution is used under pressure

32. Which of the following may be used for surface disinfectant in the dental office?
   a. iodophors
   b. ethyl alcohol
   c. isopropyl alcohol
   d. hydrogen peroxide

33. Before dental x-ray films are exposed, the treatment area must be prepared using:
   a. antiseptic
   b. aseptic techniques
   c. sterilization of critical instruments
   d. low-level disinfectant

34. Manufacturers of sterilizers (autoclaves) set them to reach a maximum steam temperature of ____ °F and pressure of ____ pounds per square inch (psi).
   a. 250, 15 to 30
   b. 350, 10 to 25
   c. 400, 25
   d. 500, 40

35. According to CDC guidelines, when transporting a biopsy specimen, it should be:
   a. placed in a flexible, leak-proof container with a plain label and marked *hazardous.*
   b. placed in a sturdy, leak-proof container labeled with a biohazard symbol.
   c. placed in an OSHA-approved container and handled only by a federally licensed handler.
   d. placed in a sterile saline solution and then in a sturdy, leak-proof container labeled with a biohazard symbol.

36. Instruments must be absolutely dry or they will rust or have an ash layer when using which type of sterilization process?
   a. chemical vapor
   b. cold sterile
   c. steam autoclave
   d. flash sterilization

37. Which of the following are considered to be semicritical instruments in radiography?
   a. the exposure button
   b. the x-ray control panel
   c. the lead apron
   d. x-ray film holding device

38. Which of the following statements is true concerning cleaning and disinfection of the dental unit and environmental surfaces?
   a. An intermediate-level disinfectant is recommended.
   b. A low-level disinfectant is recommended.
   c. EPA-registered chemical germicides labeled as both hospital disinfectants and tuberculocidals are classified as low-level disinfectants.
   d. Only high level disinfectants should be used.

39. Which method of sterilization requires good ventilation?
   a. steam under pressure
   b. cold chemical/immersion disinfection
   c. chemical vapor
   d. flash sterilization

40. Which method is used to sterilize unwrapped instruments for immediate use?
   a. steam under pressure
   b. cold chemical/immersion disinfection
   c. unsaturated chemical vapor
   d. flash sterilization

41. From the list below, select the best procedure for caring for an explorer.
   a. steam under pressure
   b. chemical disinfection
   c. sharps container
   d. spray–wipe–spray with surface disinfectant

42. From the list below, select the best procedure for caring for a mouth mirror.
   a. steam under pressure with emulsion
   b. steam under pressure without emulsion
   c. cold chemical/immersion
   d. spray–wipe–spray with surface disinfectant

43. From the list below, select the best procedure for caring for a pair of crown and collar scissors.
   a. steam under pressure with emulsion
   b. steam under pressure without emulsion
   c. cold chemical/immersion
   d. spray–wipe–spray with surface disinfectant

44. From the list below, select the best procedure for caring for a handpiece.
   a. steam under pressure with emulsion
   b. steam under pressure without emulsion
   c. cold chemical/immersion
   d. spray wipe–spray

45. From the list below, select the best procedure for caring for a saliva ejector.
   a. steam under pressure with emulsion
   b. steam under pressure without emulsion
   c. cold chemical/immersion
   d. discard

46. From the list below, select the best procedure for caring for a contaminated needle.
   a. steam under pressure with emulsion
   b. steam under pressure without emulsion
   c. sharps container
   d. discard in biohazard container

47. From the list below, select the best procedure for caring for a pair of protective glasses.
   a. steam under pressure with emulsion
   b. steam under pressure without emulsion
   c. soap, water, and disinfectant
   d. spray–wipe–spray with surface disinfectant

48. From the list below, select the best procedure for caring for medication bottles.
   a. steam under pressure with emulsion
   b. steam under pressure without emulsion
   c. discard
   d. spray–wipe–spray or wipe–wait–wipe with surface disinfectant

49. Which type of sterilization used in the dental office requires the highest temperature?
   a. steam autoclave
   b. chemical vapor
   c. dry heat sterilization
   d. chemical liquid sterilization

50. Immersion in a chemical liquid sterilant requires at least ____ hour(s) of contact time for sterilization to occur.
   a. 1
   b. 5
   c. 10
   d. 24

51. Which of the following is *not* a recommended method for sterilizing dental burs?
   a. chemical liquid sterilization
   b. steam sterilization
   c. chemical vapor sterilization
   d. flash sterilization

52. Select the ideal instrument processing area.
   a. large enough for several assistants to work at once
   b. dedicated only to instrument processing
   c. part of the treatment rooms and dental laboratory
   d. outside the dental suite

53. There are areas of the instrument processing facility that govern the workflow pattern. The processing should flow in a single loop from:
   a. dirty to sterile to storage
   b. dirty to clean to sterile to storage
   c. dirty to preclean to clean to storage
   d. dirty to preclean to clean to sterilize to storage

54. What is the purpose of a holding solution?
   a. clean instruments
   b. disinfect instruments
   c. prevent the drying of blood and debris on instruments
   d. sterilize instruments

55. The least desirable method of precleaning dental instruments is:
    a. hand scrubbing
    b. ultrasonic cleaning
    c. automated washer
    d. a holding solution

56. The ultrasonic cleaner should be cleaned and disinfected:
    a. every other day
    b. once a week
    c. once a day
    d. once every 28 days

57. After instruments have completed the cleaning cycle of the ultrasonic cleaner, they should be:
    a. bagged
    b. rinsed with water
    c. placed in the sterilizer
    d. stored

58. The ultrasonic cleaner:
    a. cleans and removes debris
    b. cleans and disinfects
    c. cleans and sterilizes
    d. prewashes

59. Why is it important to keep an MSDS for the liquid sterilant (e.g., glutaraldehyde) on file?
    a. It completes the history of all materials used in the office.
    b. It provides information on how to protect against exposure to a chemical and what to do if an exposure occurs.
    c. It updates the records for future inspections.
    d. It will prevent an exposure.

60. The process that kills disease-causing microorganisms, but not necessarily all microbial life, is called:
    a. precleaning
    b. sterilization
    c. disinfection
    d. cleaning

61. Spores of *Bacillus atrophaeus* are used to monitor which of the following types of sterilizers?
    a. steam under pressure
    b. dry heat
    c. unsaturated chemical vapor

62. Patient care instruments are categorized into various classifications. Into which classification would instruments such as surgical forceps, scalpels, bone chisels, and scalers be placed?
    a. critical
    b. semicritical
    c. noncritical

63. For which of the following is there *not* a vaccine?
    a. influenza
    b. hepatitis B
    c. tetanus
    d. strep throat

64. Select the heat sterilization method that requires good ventilation in the dental office.
    a. hot water sterilization
    b. steam under pressure
    c. chemical vapor sterilization
    d. dry-heat sterilization

65. *Legionella* bacteria can cause what type of condition in a susceptible person?
    a. liver damage
    b. pneumonia
    c. intestinal damage
    d. skin disease

66. Nosocomial infections are commonly acquired in:
    a. a dental office
    b. any type of business office
    c. a hospital or other medical facility
    d. restaurants

67. According to OSHA, the dental assistant may do which of the following before depositing a contaminated needle in a designated puncture-resistant container?
    a. recap it
    b. bend it
    c. break it
    d. cut it

68. OSHA requires a *minimum* period of training of dental personnel in which of the following areas?
    a. MSDS Standards
    b. the Hazard Communication Standard
    c. Specialty Safety Standards
    d. State Safety Standards

69. Which of the following is the goal of a sound infection control program to reduce cross-contamination?
    a. patient to work
    b. patient to office manager
    c. dental team members to other patients
    d. community health program to the dental practice

70. Which of the following statements is true as it relates to the environmental infection control in a clinical area?
    a. Change barriers daily.
    b. Avoid the use of carpet and cloth-upholstered furnishings.
    c. Use isopropyl alcohol on fixed surfaces.
    d. Avoid barriers on light handles.

71. The Organization for Safety and Asepsis Procedures (OSAP) identifies the classification of clinical touch surfaces to include which of the following?
    a. instrument trays, handpiece holders, and countertops
    b. light handles, dental unit controls, and chair switches
    c. unit master switch, fixed cabinetry, and patient records
    d. telephone, assistant stool, and fixed cabinetry

72. Which of the following is a recommended method of preventing surface contamination?
   a. Use a surface barrier.
   b. Wipe the surface with alcohol.
   c. Use an intermediate-level disinfectant.
   d. Use a high-level disinfectant.

73. What are standard precautions?
   a. the concept that considers all patients to have infections with a bloodborne pathogen
   b. the use of the same infection control procedures for all types of health care facilities
   c. the concept that considers that blood and all patient body fluids are potentially infectious
   d. the use of only infection control procedures formally approved by a government agency

74. The best time to clean and disinfect a dental prosthesis or impression that will be processed in the office laboratory is:
   a. after it has had time to dry
   b. after it is in the laboratory
   c. when it is convenient
   d. as soon as possible after removal from the patient's mouth

75. A victim who immediately feels the effects of a chemical spill with symptoms of dizziness, headache, nausea, and vomiting, is experiencing:
   a. chronic chemical toxicity
   b. acute chemical toxicity
   c. chemical resistance
   d. mild exposure

76. _____ is considered regulated waste and requires special disposal.
   a. Human tissue
   b. Food
   c. Saliva-soaked gauze
   d. Used anesthetic cartridge

77. Repeated exposure to chemicals at low levels for extended periods of time can result in liver disease or brain disorders that are examples of:
   a. chronic chemical toxicity
   b. acute chemical toxicity
   c. terminal chemical toxicity
   d. median chemical toxicity

78. How often should a dental assistant or office safety supervisor check the contents of the emergency kit to determine that the contents are in place and within the expiration date?
   a. weekly
   b. monthly
   c. biannually
   d. annually

79. The floor in the entry to the dental office was wet. A patient slipped on the floor during entry to the office. There was no signage to include a potential slippery floor. In this case, the office owner:
   a. is responsible for providing signage for potential dangerous situations
   b. is not held liable because the entry is not part of the clinical area
   c. is not held liable because the patient should have been able to see the wet area because he or she was not legally blind
   d. does not fall under such regulations because of the number of employees

80. Wastes are classified as hazardous if they are:
    a. ignitable
    b. ingestible
    c. ultrasonic
    d. plastic

81. All waste containers that hold potentially infectious materials must:
    a. have a red bag
    b. be labeled with the biohazard symbol
    c. have special disposal
    d. be labeled as infectious waste

82. Scrap dental amalgam should be collected and stored in:
    a. a designated dry, airtight container
    b. an airtight container under a disinfectant
    c. an airtight container under water or photographer fixer
    d. a clear glass jar

83. Which government agency enforces the disposal of regulated waste?
    a. OSHA
    b. EPA
    c. CDC
    d. FDA

84. Which of the following does the OSHA Hazard Communications Standard require employers to do?
    a. Submit annual drug test results of all employees.
    b. Maintain accurate and thorough employee tax records.
    c. Submit annual urinalysis results of all employees.
    d. Tell employees about the identity and hazards of chemicals in the workplace.

85. Which of the following is the dental staff required to have available and know the location of in the event of a heart attack or closed or blocked airway?
    a. crash cart
    b. oxygen
    c. IV stimulants
    d. patient's medications

86. Which of the following is *not* a requirement of hazard communication training?
    a. hazards of chemicals and proper handling of chemicals
    b. the availability and access of MSDS to all staff
    c. an explanation of the labeling of hazardous chemicals
    d. waivers of hepatitis C vaccinations

87. A dental health care worker transfers a small amount of glass ionomer cement into a smaller container for use on a patient at chairside. A new label must be placed on that container if:
    a. more material is required during the course of treating that patient
    b. the chemical material is not used up at the conclusion of an 8-hour work shift
    c. the patient recently tested positive for HIV
    d. no MSDS can be found on file for that material

88. Hazard communication training must be provided:
   a. for all new employees at the beginning of employment
   b. any time a new hazardous material is introduced into the office
   c. biannually
   d. quarterly

89. Which of the following is an unsafe practice when recapping the needle?
   a. a one-handed scoop method
   b. a mechanical device specifically designed to hold the needle for recapping
   c. any safety feature that is fixed, provides a barrier between the assistant's hands and the needle after use, and allows the assistant's hands to remain behind the needle
   d. a two-handed scoop method for maximum control

90. Which of the following is *not* considered a "sharp"?
   a. metal matrix band
   b. metal matrix retainer
   c. orthodontic wire
   d. needle

91. Flushing the water lines of the dental unit relates to:
   a. temporarily trapping debris from the water lines
   b. bringing a fresh supply of warm chlorinated water into the dental unit
   c. reduction of microbial count in the water
   d. removing biofilm from the lines

92. The ADA, OSAP, and CDC recommend that dental assistants flush the dental unit waterlines:
   a. for 30 seconds each morning and again at the end of the day
   b. for 30 seconds each morning and between patients
   c. for 60 seconds each morning and 30 seconds after treating an HIV-infected patient
   d. for 30 seconds each hour of the day

93. Shortly after donning the required PPE, a dental health care worker notices the following symptoms: watering eyes, nasal congestion, sneezing, coughing, wheezing, shortness of breath, and even dizziness. This person may be experiencing which type of reaction?
   a. immediate hypersensitivity (type I)
   b. delayed hypersensitivity (type IV)
   c. intermediate hypersensitivity (type III)
   d. irritant dermatitis (ID)

94. Which of the following are the recommended five parts of the Hazard Communication Standard?
   a. written program, inventory of hazardous chemicals, inventory of dental instruments, proper labeling of containers, employee training
   b. written program, inventory of hazardous chemicals, MSDS for every chemical, proper labeling of containers, employee training
   c. written records of staff health histories, inventory of hazardous chemicals, MSDS for every chemical, proper labeling of containers, employee training
   d. written program, inventory of hazardous chemicals, MSDS for every chemical, staff hair or urinalysis reports, employee training

95. Select the statement that is *not* true.
    a. AIDS is a worldwide problem.
    b. HIV causes AIDS.
    c. HIV is transmitted through casual contact.
    d. HIV testing is recommended 6 months after the last possible exposure to HIV.

96. Switching to instruments with large, round diameters and contra-angled shanks may _____ the symptoms associated with carpal tunnel syndrome.
    a. help reduce
    b. exacerbate
    c. have little effect on
    d. have no effect on

97. Which of the following activities should be avoided during the use of nitrous oxide during conscious sedation?
    a. Maintain conversation with the patient.
    b. Use dental dam when applicable.
    c. Use a scavenger system.
    d. Secure the patient's mask.

98. Distillation of water is a _____ process that may remove volatile chemicals, endotoxins, and some microorganisms.
    a. sterilization
    b. reverse osmosis
    c. purification
    d. radiation

99. Which of the following statements is true regarding the use of biohazard warning labels?
    a. The label is fluorescent orange or red-orange.
    b. The word *biohazard* is placed only on labels for sharps.
    c. A label must be placed on all dental office waste.
    d. White or green bags may be substituted for labels.

100. OSHA requires the use of standard precautions for _____.
    a. HIV-infected or AIDS patients
    b. potentially disease-infected patients
    c. patients not of record
    d. all patients

Answer Keys and Rationales

TEST 1

General Chairside

1. The position of the body standing erect with the feet together and the arms hanging at the sides with the palms facing forward is referred to as the _____ position.
   b. The anatomic position refers to the body when it is in a vertical position with the face and the palms of the hands facing forward. A resting or postural position is not a term used in anatomic descriptions, and the supine position places a person on the back with the face up.
   CAT: Chairside Dental Procedures

2. In the illustration shown, Dr. Curtis was assisted by Debbie May Ross to complete operative treatment for this patient. What required data are missing from the chart?
   d. The space for the file number was left blank. To be a legal document, a number or "NA" for "not applicable" should be inserted. The date of the appointment and the initials of the dentist and the dental assistant performing the treatment must also be included.
   CAT: Collection and Recording of Clinical Data

3. The examination technique in which the examiner uses his or her fingers to feel for size, texture, and consistency of hard and soft tissue is called:
   b. Palpation is the examination technique in which the examiner uses the fingers to feel for the size, texture, and consistency of hard and soft tissue. Determination is the act of making a decision. Inspection is a visual observation. Assessment is the process of gathering information, not a specific technique.
   CAT: Collection and Recording of Clinical Data

4. Which type of consent is given when a patient enters a dentist's office?
   b. Implied consent refers to the duties or actions that flow automatically for the relationship between the patient and the dental professional. The patient gives implied consent when he or she enters the dentist's office, at least for the dental exam. This is not informed consent, which demands more disclosure on the part of the provider about the care given a patient.
   CAT: Office Operations

5. Consent is:
   b. Consent is voluntary, and it is given by a patient when he or she agrees to accept what is planned or done for him or her by another person. To give consent, a person must be 18 years of age or older.
   CAT: Office Operations

6. A patient's chart that denotes a congenital absence of some or all of the teeth would indicate:
   d. Anodontia can be broken down to *an*, meaning without, and *odontia*, meaning teeth. Micrognathia is a condition in which the jaw is undersized. Ankylosis is fixation of a tooth resulting from fusion of the cementum and alveolar bone. Macrognathia refers to the condition of abnormally large jaws.
   CAT: Collection and Recording of Clinical Data

7. The tooth-numbering system that begins with the maxillary right third molar as tooth #1 and ends with the mandibular right third molar as tooth #32 is the _____ system.
   a. The Universal numbering system begins with the maxillary right third molar as tooth #1 and ends with the mandibular right third molar as tooth #32. The other

systems use either brackets or other numeric patterns to denote tooth numbering.
CAT: Collection and Recording of Clinical Data

8. An abbreviation used in the progress notes or chart to indicate a mesioocclusobuccal restoration is:
   d. Each surface is given an initial, and in the naming of this restoration, the surfaces are in the sequence of mesial, occlusal, and buccal—thus, MOB.
   CAT: Collection and Recording of Clinical Data

9. A developmental abnormality characterized by the complete bonding of two adjacent teeth caused by irregular growth is:
   b. Fusion involves the entire length of two teeth to form one large tooth. Concrescence is a condition of teeth in which the cementum overlying the roots of at least two teeth joins together. Germination is the incomplete splitting of a single tooth germ. Ankylosis is fixation of a tooth resulting from fusion of the cementum and alveolar bone.
   CAT: Collection and Recording of Clinical Data

10. A(n) _____ tooth is any tooth that is prevented from reaching its normal position in the mouth by tissue, bone, or another tooth.
    b. An impacted tooth is one that is so positioned in the jaw bone that eruption is not possible.
    CAT: Collection and Recording of Clinical Data

11. An oral habit consisting of involuntary gnashing, grinding, and clenching of the teeth is:
    b. Bruxism is the process of grinding the teeth. Erosion is the loss of tooth surface caused by a chemical process. Abrasion and attrition are both mechanical processes of wearing away of the tooth surface.
    CAT: Collection and Recording of Clinical Data

12. A horizontal or transverse plane divides the body into:
    a. When a body is divided horizontally, it will produce an upper and a lower portion or superior and inferior portions.
    CAT: Collection and Recording of Clinical Data

13. The cells associated with bone formation are known as:
    d. An osteoblast is a cell of mesodermal origin that is concerned with the formation of bone.
    CAT: Collection and Recording of Clinical Data

14. The air/water syringe should be flushed for _____ at beginning and end of each day.
    b. Flushing for 2 minutes at the beginning and end of the day clears the water lines. Thirty seconds is not long enough, and 5 or 30 minutes is too long a time and not necessary.
    CAT: Chairside Dental Procedures

15. One of the functions of the paranasal sinuses is to:
    b. One of the functions of the paranasal sinuses is to aid in warming respired air. There is no relationship between sinuses and digestion, smelling, or absorbing bacteria.
    CAT: Collection and Recording of Clinical Data

16. The air/water syringe should be flushed for at least _____ between patients.
    a. Flushing for 30 seconds between patients is sufficient to clean a water line. Three, 5, or 30 minutes is too long a time and not necessary.
    CAT: Chairside Dental Procedures

17. Which zone corresponds to the 4 o'clock to 7 o'clock region?
    a. Using the clock concept, the 4 to 7 o'clock region is the transfer region. There is no activity zone. The assisting or assistant's zone is the 2 to 4 o'clock region. The static zone is between the 12 and 2 o'clock region.
    CAT: Chairside Dental Procedures

18. A 10-year-old patient would likely have which of the following teeth?
    a. At the age of 10 years, a child could have the permanent mandibular central and lateral incisors, primary second molars, permanent mandibular canines, and permanent first molars but would not yet have the permanent premolars or second molars.
    CAT: Chairside Dental Procedures

19. What is the average range of the body's oral resting temperature?
    d. The normal adult body temperature is considered to be 98. 6° F but may range between 97.6° F and 99° F.
    CAT: Collection and Recording of Clinical Data

20. In dentistry the acronym HVE represents:
    a. An acronym is a word formed from the initial letters of a name. HVE is derived from high-volume evacuation.
    CAT: Chairside Dental Procedures

21. The primary step in preventing a medical emergency is to be certain the patient has _____ before treatment is begun.
    c. It is necessary to obtain a complete medical history for each patient and update this health history at regular intervals. Without an accurate and updated health history, the dental professional is unaware of potential health risks.
    CAT: Prevention and Management of Emergencies

22. What are the symptoms a patient would display when experiencing a cerebrovascular accident?
    a. Some of the symptoms of a cerebrovascular accident, also known as a stroke, include paralysis, speech problems, and vision problems. Hunger, sweating, and mood change are symptoms of hypoglycemia. Itching, erythema, and hives are symptoms of an allergic reaction. Coughing, wheezing, and an increased pulse rate are symptoms of an asthma attack.
    CAT: Prevention and Management of Emergencies

23. The most current adult basic life support protocol (CAB) is an acronym for:
    a. Compressions, airway, and breathing are the steps to be taken when providing basic life support.
    CAT: Prevention and Management of Emergencies

24. The most frequently used substance in a medical emergency is:
    b. Glucose, epinephrine, and ammonia inhalants are included in an emergency kit, but oxygen is the most frequently used drug in a medical emergency.
    CAT: Prevention and Management of Emergencies

25. The leading cause of heart attack is:
    d. Coronary artery disease, also known as coronary heart disease, is a narrowing of the blood vessels that supply blood and oxygen to the heart. Rheumatic fever, if left untreated, can affect the heart valves but is not a leading cause of heart attack. Valvular heart disease and infective endocarditis also affect the heart but are not leading causes of heart attack.
    CAT: Prevention and Management of Emergencies

26. Which of the following is precipitated by stress and anxiety; may manifest in rapid, shallow breathing, lightheadedness, a rapid heartbeat, and a panic-stricken appearance; and is treated by having the patient breathe into a paper bag or cupped hands?
    b. When a patient is anxious or apprehensive, he or she may display rapid, shallow breathing; lightheadedness; a rapid heartbeat; and a panic-stricken appearance. The patient is treated by breathing into a paper bag or cupped hands to increase the carbon dioxide supply and to restore the proper oxygen and carbon dioxide levels in the blood.
    CAT: Prevention and Management of Emergencies

27. While you are providing dental treatment for a patient in her third trimester of pregnancy, the patient suddenly feels dizzy and short of breath. How should the patient be repositioned in the dental chair?
    b. Tilted to the left side keeps the aorta and inferior vena cava from being compressed by the uterus. In a subsupine position, the patient's head would be lower than the feet, making the situation worse. Parallel is equivalent to a supine position, and in both positions, the weight of the fetus and uterus bears down on the major vessels, restricting the patient's blood flow to the heart.
    CAT: Prevention and Management of Emergencies

28. To ensure that a medical emergency is observed immediately, it is important for the dental assistant to:

c. Because the dentist is concentrating on treatment in the oral cavity, the dental assistant needs to observe the patient throughout the procedure to note any changes in behavior or vital signs that would indicate potential medical complications.
CAT: **Prevention and Management of Emergencies**

29. What are the symptoms a patient would display when experiencing hypoglycemia?

b. Hunger, sweating, and mood change are symptoms of hypoglycemia. Symptoms of cerebrovascular accident include paralysis, speech problems, and vision problems. Itching, erythema, and hives are symptoms of an allergic reaction. Coughing, wheezing, and an increased pulse rate are symptoms of an asthma attack.
CAT: **Prevention and Management of Emergencies**

30. In relation to ergonomics in a dental business office, there are how many classifications of motion?

b. There are five classifications of motion, which include class I: fingers–only movement; class II: fingers and wrist movement; class III: fingers, wrist, and elbow movement; class IV: fingers, wrist, elbow, and shoulder movement; and class V: arm extension and twisting of the torso.
CAT: **Chairside Dental Procedures**

31. The distance between the operator's face and the patient's oral cavity should be approximately _____ inches.

c. Although an average, 16 inches is the optimal distance. Six or 10 inches is too close and creates stress on the operator's neck. A distance of 24 inches is too far, and the operator may not have a clear field of vision.
CAT: **Chairside Dental Procedures**

32. While positioned in the dental assisting stool, the dental assistant should rest his or her feet:

b. The dental assisting stool is designed so the assistant's feet can rest on the tubular bar. If the dental assistant's stool is at the correct height, the assistant would not be able to reach the floor. The legs of the stool support the tubular bar but are not the ideal location for placement of the feet.
CAT: **Chairside Dental Procedures**

33. Which of the following medical conditions is considered a contraindication for nitrous oxide analgesia?

a. The effects of nitrous oxide analgesia may increase negative reactions in a person with severe emotional disturbances. High blood pressure, epilepsy, and diabetes are unaffected by nitrous oxide analgesia.
CAT: **Prevention and Management of Emergencies**

34. Motion economy is the concept that encourages the dental health care worker to:

b. To conserve energy and increase productivity, motion economy is used to decrease the number and length of motions at chairside.
CAT: **Chairside Dental Procedures**

35. Which of the following instruments would be found on a prophylaxis tray setup?

c. A scaler is used to remove calculus from the teeth and would be on a prophylaxis tray setup. A spoon excavator and burnisher would be on an amalgam tray setup, and a pocket marker is used to mark tissue for a gingivectomy and would be on a periodontal surgery tray setup.
CAT: **Chairside Dental Procedures**

36. The lowest level of Maslow's hierarchy of needs is:

a. Physiologic needs are requirements for human survival and are the lowest level on Maslow's hierarchy. Security is the second level, social is the third level, esteem is the fourth level, and self–actualization is the fifth and top level.
CAT: **Patient Education and Oral Health Management**

37. Which of the following should be done if the patient has thick, heavy saliva that adheres to the prophylaxis cup during the polishing procedure?

b. The HVE tip, when placed close to polishing cup, will prevent the thick, heavy saliva from

adhering to the rubber cup, making it easier to polish the teeth. A saliva ejector is not strong enough to remove this heavy saliva.
CAT: Chairside Dental Procedures

38. Plaster of Paris and dental stone are examples of:

c. Gypsum products include plaster of Paris and dental stone. These are products used to pour into a dental impression. Impression materials are used to take dental impressions. Impression trays hold the impression material, and intermediary materials are temporary materials.
CAT: Chairside Dental Materials (Preparation, Manipulation, Application)

39. The portion of a bridge that replaces the missing tooth is called a(n):

c. The portion of the bridge that replaces the missing tooth is called the pontic, and the portion that is used for support or retention of the fixed prosthesis is the abutment.
CAT: Lab Materials and Procedures

40. Which of the following instruments would be used to measure the depth of the gingival sulcus?

a. The periodontal probe is designed with calibrations on the tip end to enable the operator to measure the depth of the gingival sulcus during routine examinations. The other instruments can identify dental anomalies but are not capable of measurement.
CAT: Chairside Dental Procedures

41. Which of the following instruments is used to scale an area specific deep periodontal pocket?

a. A Gracey curette is a site-specific scaling instrument. It is used for a specific area of the tooth, such as the mesial or distal surface, depending on the type of Gracey. The sickle and hoe scalers are not site specific. A spoon excavator is not a scaling instrument.
CAT: Chairside Dental Procedures

42. The HVE system is used:

b. The HVE system is designed to remove large volumes of fluid and debris from the mouth during all operative and surgical

procedures. The saliva ejector is a slow-speed evacuator and is not capable of removing debris from the mouth.
CAT: Chairside Dental Procedures

43. Which of the following instruments can be used to invert the rubber dam?

b. Although dental floss enables the operator to move the rubber dam into position at the interproximal surfaces of the tooth, the spoon excavator with a curved blade enables the operator to smoothly invert the rubber dam into the gingival sulcus. The explorer has a sharp, pointed tip and could tear the dam and damage the soft tissue.
CAT: Chairside Dental Procedures

44. If treatment is to be performed on tooth #13, the clamp is placed on which tooth placement?

a. The general rule for rubber dam placement during an operative procedure is to place the clamp on the tooth distal to the last tooth being treated and then isolate the tooth being treated and the two teeth mesial to this tooth.
CAT: Chairside Dental Procedures

45. You are assisting a right-handed operator in a procedure performed on the patient's left side. The HVE tip and A/W syringe are being used. The operator signals for a transfer. You must:

b. For the assistant to pick up a new instrument to be transferred, it will be necessary to transfer the A/W syringe to the right hand, retain the HVE tip in the right hand, and pick up the new instrument to be transferred.
CAT: Chairside Dental Procedures

46. Which of the following is the correct statement regarding the seating position of the operator?

a. The operator's thighs are parallel to the floor to give the least amount of stress to the operator's back and hip area. Sitting on the edge of the chair or placing feet on the chair legs produces stress to the operator's body. The operator can work from several clock positions depending on the area of the mouth the operator is working on.
CAT: Chairside Dental Procedures

47. When placing the amalgam into the preparation for a 31DO restoration, the first increment should be placed into the:
   b. The first increment is placed into the proximal box because this is the most difficult area to gain access. After the amalgam reaches the pulpal floor region, the amalgam can be packed into this area more easily.
   CAT: Chairside Dental Procedures

48. Which of the following instruments would be used to grasp tissue or bone fragments during a surgical procedure?
   a. The hemostat is a holding device that enables a person to grasp and clamp the tissue or material in place without fear of slippage. It is used often in surgery to grasp small tissue fragments to remove them from the region. Locking pliers do not have the grasping capability of hemostats, and both of the other instruments are not used to grasp materials or tissues.
   CAT: Chairside Dental Procedures

49. Which of the following is the common choice in providing for retention in a cavity preparation?
   d. The small round bur, such as a no. ½, is a desirable bur to make a retentive groove. It forms a rounded surface on the cavity preparation floor to enable the material to lock in place.
   CAT: Chairside Dental Procedures

50. What type of matrix is used for an anterior esthetic restoration?
   a. A celluloid strip will not stick to the material used in an anterior esthetic restoration. A metal or contoured matrix band is used for amalgam restorations. A finishing strip is used to smooth an anterior esthetic restoration after it has set.
   CAT: Chairside Dental Procedures

51. When placing a composite restoration on the buccal cervical of tooth #30, which is the choice of matrix?
   b. The class V composite matrix is desirable because it is shaped in an oval form to replicate the shape of the cervical area of the tooth.
   CAT: Chairside Dental Procedures

52. The most common form of anesthesia used in operative dentistry is:
   a. Local anesthesia is used most often in operative dentistry. The other forms of anesthesia are used in specific situations but are not used commonly in operative dentistry.
   CAT: Chairside Dental Procedures

53. For dental professionals, the safest allowable amount of N$_2$O is _____ parts per million.
   a. For dental professionals, the safest allowable amount of N$_2$O is 50 parts per million. More than this amount in the dental environment may cause adverse effects.
   CAT: Prevention and Management of Emergencies

54. Which of the following medical conditions is a contraindication to using a vasoconstrictor in the local anesthesia during operative treatment?
   b. A vasoconstrictor tightens blood vessels and reduces blood flow. A person with a recent heart attack had that attack because of blood vessel restriction. A vasoconstrictor may compound the problem. Diabetes and epilepsy are not affected by a vasoconstrictor. Although a vasoconstrictor can cross the placenta, it is not a danger to the mother or fetus.
   CAT: Prevention and Management of Emergencies

55. _____ is frequently used on the mandibular teeth and is injected near a major nerve that anesthetizes the entire area served by that nerve branch.
   a. Block anesthesia is the type of injection frequently required for most mandibular teeth and is injected near a major nerve. Block anesthesia numbs the entire area served by the nerve.
   CAT: Chairside Dental Procedures

56. Nitrous oxide oxygen administration always begins and ends with:
   b. The patient is given 100% oxygen at the beginning of nitrous oxide administration to assist the dentist in determining the

patient's tidal volume. Oxygenation at the end of the procedure helps to prevent a feeling of light headedness.
CAT: Chairside Dental Procedures

57. When there is not enough teeth structure to hold a prosthetic crown, a _____ is used to aid in retention.
    b. A core buildup consists of material (amalgam or composite) that is designed to replace missing tooth structure to aid in supporting a crown. A matrix band is used during the placement of amalgam. A celluloid strip is used during composite placement. A retention pin supports amalgam or composite material when extensive tooth structure has been lost.
    CAT: Chairside Dental Procedures

58. The tray setup in the photograph is used to:
    d. The key instruments on this tray are the ligature ties, director, hemostat, and ligature cutter, which are all related to the placement and removal of ligature ties. There are no bands or separators available.
    CAT: Chairside Dental Procedures

59. To control swelling after a surgical procedure, the patient should be instructed to:
    a. Edema or swelling can best be reduced or kept to a minimum if the patient is directed to place a cold pack in a cycle of 20 minutes on and 20 minutes off for the first 24 hours. Heat is contraindicated for the reduction of swelling.
    CAT: Patient Education and Oral Health Management

60. The painful condition that can result from the premature loss of a blood clot after a tooth extraction is known as:
    b. Alveolitis is the premature loss of a blood clot after extraction. Periodontitis is an inflammatory disease affecting the periodontium. Hemostasis is the stopping of bleeding or blood flow through a blood vessel. Gingivitis is a reversible inflammatory disease affecting the periodontium that may progress to periodontitis if left untreated.
    CAT: Patient Education and Oral Health Management

61. It may take _____ to complete a dental implant procedure.
    c. Depending on the complexity of the procedure and healing, it will take between 3 and 9 months to complete a dental implant procedure.
    CAT: Patient Education and Oral Health Management

62. A metal frame that is placed under the periosteum and on top of the bone is called a(n):
    b. The prefix *sub* means "under" or "beneath" and thus identifies this answer as the subperiosteal implant because the metal frame is placed under the periosteum
    CAT: Chairside Dental Procedures

63. The natural rubber material used to obturate the pulp canal after treatment is completed is called:
    b. Gutta–percha is a natural rubber material used to obturate the pulpal canal after treatment has been completed. Neither hydrogen peroxide nor glass ionomer is used to obturate the canal.
    CAT: Chairside Dental Materials (Preparation, Manipulation, Application)

64. In this photograph, which instrument is a barbed broach?
    a. The photograph in **a** illustrates the barbs that appear on a barbed broach.
    CAT: Chairside Dental Procedures

65. A common solution used for irrigation during the debridement procedure in endodontic treatment is:
    c. Sodium hypochlorite, commonly referred to as bleach, is the common solution used for irrigating a canal during debridement. Sterile water and salt solutions are not used.
    CAT: Chairside Dental Procedures

66. The incisional periodontal surgical procedure that does not remove tissues but pushes away the underlying tooth roots and alveolar bone is known as:
    c. In incisional surgery, also known as periodontal flap surgery or simply flap surgery, the tissues are not removed but are

pushed away form the underlying tooth roots and alveolar bone.
CAT: Chairside Dental Procedures

67. According to recent studies, periodontal disease is associated with an increased risk of developing which of the following conditions?
    c. Recent studies indicate periodontal disease may increase the inflammation level throughout the body, thereby increasing the risk for cardiovascular disease.
    CAT: Patient Education and Oral Health Management

68. The _____ is an instrument that resembles a large spoon and is used to debride the interior of the socket to remove diseased tissue and abscesses.
    c. The surgical curette has two spoon-like tips that aid in debriding or cleaning out the interior surface of the socket after the removal of a tooth.
    CAT: Chairside Dental Procedures

69. From the instruments shown here, select the curette.
    d. The photograph in **d** has two ends with spoon-like tips that are characteristic of a surgical curette.
    CAT: Chairside Dental Procedures

70. Coronal polishing is a technique used to remove_____ from tooth surfaces.
    c. Only plaque can be removed with coronal polishing. Calculus and cement are removed by scaling. Only extrinsic stain can be removed with polishing.
    CAT: Chairside Dental Procedures

71. What terms are used to classify stain by location?
    b. Extrinsic staining is on the exterior surface of the teeth. Intrinsic staining is on the interior surface of teeth. *Exogenous* and *endogenous* are terms associated with disease. Exogenous means it is externally caused rather than endogenous, resulting from conditions within the organism.
    CAT: Patient Education and Oral Health Management

72. The purpose of using disclosing solution is to _____
    b. Disclosing solution is used to visualize plaque. An explorer is used to identify calculus. Disclosing solution does not desensitize tooth structure or destroy bacteria.
    CAT: Patient Education and Oral Health Management

73. The first step in placing dental sealants is to _____ the surface.
    c. Before a sealant can be placed, the tooth surface must be adequately cleaned.
    CAT: Chairside Dental Procedures

74. Enamel that has been etched has the appearance of being:
    a. When the enamel has been etched appropriately, it will have a chalky appearance and will not be shiny, wet, or slightly discolored.
    CAT: Chairside Dental Procedures

75. Which of the following medical emergencies would be treated with a bronchodilator?
    c. A bronchodilator is a substance that dilates the bronchi and bronchioles, thereby increasing air flow to the lungs during an asthma attack. No medication is given during an epileptic seizure. A cerebrovascular accident (stroke) is treated by attaining immediate medical assistance. A hypoglycemic incident is treated by administering glucose to the person.
    CAT: Prevention and Management of Emergencies

76. The isolation of multiple anterior teeth requires the dental dam be placed _____.
    c. To adequately isolate the anterior region when more than one tooth is being treated, it is recommended that teeth from first premolar to first premolar be isolated. By isolating from first premolar to first premolar, stability to the rubber dam will exist during isolation.
    CAT: Chairside Dental Procedures

77. During a dental procedure, the dental assistant's stool is _____ the operator's stool.
    b. The dental assistant's stool is higher than the operator's stool for optimum visibility

by the dental assistant. An assistant's stool that is lower than, the same height as, or even with the operator's stool does not allow optimum visibility and can put stress on the dental assistant's body.
CAT: **Chairside Dental Procedures**

78. Gingival retraction cord is placed _____ the crown preparation is completed and is removed _____ the final impression is taken.
    d. after, before. Before taking the final impression after the crown preparation is completed, retraction cord is placed into the gingival sulcus to enable retraction of the soft tissue. The impression will more adequately include the cervical margin of the preparation.
    CAT: **Chairside Dental Procedures**

79. A _____ is an orthodontic _____ that is a custom appliance made of rubber or pliable acrylic that fits over the patient's dentition after orthodontic treatment.
    d. The Hawley appliance is the most commonly used removable custom-made appliance that is used as a positioner. It is worn to passively retain the teeth in their new position after the removal of the fixed appliances.
    CAT: **Chairside Dental Procedures**

80. This tray setup is for:
    b. The setup includes elastomeric ties, hemostat, and orthodontic scaler, all instruments used in placing and removing elastomeric ties. No bands, arch wires, or separators are present.
    CAT: **Chairside Dental Procedures**

81. Instrument "A" in the photograph is used to:
    b. The instrument is a band seater. When the patient bites gently onto it, it aids the operator in forcing the band down onto approximately the middle third of the tooth.
    CAT: **Chairside Dental Procedures**

82. A(n) _____ is used to provide interproximal space for inserting an orthodontic band.
    b. The instrument is a band seater. When the patient bites gently onto it, it aids the

operator in forcing the band down onto approximately the middle third of the tooth.
CAT: **Chairside Dental Procedures**

83. Which of the following is a rotary device used with discs or wheels?
    d. Only the mandrel is a rotary device. A bur is used to cut tooth structure. An ultrasonic is a handpiece used to remove calculus. A prophy angle is a device placed on a slow-speed handpiece to polish teeth.
    CAT: **Chairside Dental Procedures**

84. When instructing a patient about treatment for angular cheilitis, where would the dental assistant tell the patient to place the topical antibiotic?
    c. Angular cheilitis is an inflammatory lesion at the labial commissure (corner of the mouth).
    CAT: **Patient Education and Oral Health Management**

85. When describing a superficial infection caused by a yeast-like fungus to a patient, what would you call this condition?
    c. Candidiasis is an infection caused by a group of yeast. Leukoplakia is a term used to describe patches on the tongue, in the mouth, or on the inside of the cheek that occur in response to long-term irritation. Lichen planus is an inflammatory condition that can affect the skin and mucous membranes caused by an abnormal immune response.
    CAT: **Patient Education and Oral Health Management**

86. Which instrument would be used to remove the right mandibular first molar?
    a. The larger beaks will enable the operator to grasp the molar more readily than the other forceps, which are used for an anterior tooth.
    CAT: **Chairside Dental Procedures**

87. Which instrument would be used to remove the right maxillary second molar?
    a. The forceps in B and C are both used for the mandible because their beaks are at nearly

right angles to the handles. The forceps in A are for the maxillary molar. Their beaks are more nearly parallel to the handles and enable the operator to use them on the maxilla.
CAT: Chairside Dental Procedures

88. Which of the following instruments would be used to remove a metal matrix band after carving an amalgam restoration?
   d. Cotton forceps are used to grasp the metal matrix for removal. A shepherd's hook explorer, rubber dam forceps, and acorn burnisher may be used during an amalgam restoration but are not associated with a matrix band.
   CAT: Chairside Dental Procedures

89. When a tooth is avulsed, it has:
   b. An avulsed tooth is a tooth that has been forcibly detached.
   CAT: Chairside Dental Procedures

90. An automated external defibrillator (AED) is used for what medical emergency?
   a. An AED is a portable electronic device that can reestablish an effective rhythm to a person who has had sudden cardiac arrest.
   CAT: Prevention and Management of Emergencies

91. One of the characteristics that allows gold to be one of the most compatible restorative materials in the oral environment is the ability to:
   a. Resisting tarnish means the gold does not become dulled or discolored. That is a desirable quality. Trituration is associated with the mixing of amalgam. If a metal is corrosive, that is a negative quality. Producing allergens is also a negative quality.
   CAT: Chairside Dental Materials (Preparation, Manipulation, Application)

92. A dental restorative material that is applied to a tooth or teeth while the material is pliable and can be adapted, carved, and finished is classified as:
   a. A direct restoration is one that is placed and carved in the tooth during a single appointment. An indirect restoration requires an impression of the prepared tooth. Then a restoration such as a crown,

bridge, or onlay is made outside the mouth and cemented into the tooth at another appointment or later time.
CAT: Chairside Dental Materials (Preparation, Manipulation, Application)

93. Which of these would have the least dimensional stability?
   c. Alginate hydrocolloid is subject to syneresis and imbibition because of the water content of the product. Thus, the dimensional stability of the material is very low.
   CAT: Chairside Dental Materials (Preparation, Manipulation, Application)

94. The conventional or traditional composites, which contain the largest filler particles and provide the greatest strength, are known as:
   d. Macrofilled composites contain the largest of the filler particles, providing the greatest strength but resulting in a duller, rougher surface. Macrofilled composites are used in areas where greater strength is required to resist fracture.
   CAT: Chairside Dental Materials (Preparation, Manipulation, Application)

95. If a light-bodied impression catalyst is mixed with a heavy-bodied impression base, the resultant mix might:
   b. The bases and catalysts of each consistency are chemically manufactured to work with the matched base or catalyst. If the base and catalyst is interchanged with the consistency tubes, the end result will not be accurate.
   CAT: Chairside Dental Materials (Preparation, Manipulation, Application)

96. Addition of cold water to an alginate mix will cause the setting time to be:
   a. When cooler temperature water is used, it will take the mix longer to set; thus, the setting time is increased.
   CAT: Chairside Dental Materials (Preparation, Manipulation, Application)

97. Select two terms that describe the purpose and consistency of a dental cement used for the final seating of a porcelain fused-to-metal crown.
   d. The final seating of porcelain fused to metal crown requires a cement base

that is of luting or primary consistency, which strings for about 1 inch. The purpose of seating the crown is for final cementation.
CAT: Chairside Dental Materials (Preparation, Manipulation, Application)

98. Which of the following is a noble metal?
   d. Palladium is a noble metal. Tin, iron, and zinc are base metals.
   CAT: Lab Materials and Procedures

99. The purpose of calcium hydroxide in a cavity preparation is to:
   b. Calcium hydroxide irritates the tooth to help form reparative dentin.
   CAT: Chairside Dental Materials (Preparation, Manipulation, Application)

100. The advantage of using a glass ionomer as a restorative material is that it:
   b. Fluoride release is a primary characteristic of glass ionomers and thus makes it a desirable restorative material.
   CAT: Chairside Dental Materials (Preparation, Manipulation, Application)

101. A custom tray is constructed to fit the mouth of a specific patient and is used to _____, _____, and _____.
   b. When a custom tray is designed for a patient, it will adapt to the patient's mouth, fit around any anomalies, and reduce the amount of impression material needed.
   CAT: Lab Materials and Procedures

102. Which form of gypsum product is commonly used for making diagnostic models?
   a. Plaster is the most porous of the gypsum products and is cost effective for use in the construction of diagnostic models.
   CAT: Lab Materials and Procedures

103. When taking impressions, the next step after seating the patient and placing the patient napkin is to:
   c. Before taking impressions, the patient must be informed of the procedure and the process explained so that there is complete cooperation.
   CAT: Lab Materials and Procedures

104. Which of the following instruments is used to cut soft tissue during a tooth extraction?
   c. A scalpel is a small, sharp-bladed instrument used for cutting tissue during surgery.
   CAT: Chairside Dental Procedures

105. Vital information on a registration form includes the _____ of person responsible for the account.
   a. Vital information about the patient includes name, address, and contact telephone numbers. Military service, type of discharge, race, citizenship, national origin, height, weight, and a picture of the patient are irrelevant or illegal information to obtain about a patient.
   CAT: Office Operations

106. Financial arrangements for dental treatment should be made:
   c. Good business practice mandates that financial arrangements must be made before beginning the treatment for the patient.
   CAT: Office Operations

107. _____ is the amount the dental assistant takes home after all deductions are made.
   b. Net pay is the amount the earner receives in the payroll check. This amount equals the amount of the gross pay minus all deductions.
   CAT: Office Operations

108. _____ is another name for the Social Security funds deducted from an employee's pay.
   b. Federal Insurance Contributions Act (FICA), commonly known as Social Security, is the amount the employer is required to deduct from the employee's gross income.
   CAT: Office Operations

109. Which of these is an expendable item used in the dental office?
   c. An expendable item is a single-use item and is discarded after the single use.
   CAT: Office Operations

110. Which is a capital item in a dental office?
   c. A capital item is one of great cost, generally more than $1000, and is reused for several years.
   CAT: Office Operations

111. Oxygen should be stored:
  b. Oxygen tanks are always stored upright and secured tightly in place.
  CAT: Office Operations

112. An office system that tracks patients' follow-up visits for an oral prophylaxis is a(n):
  c. A recall system is used to recall patients to the office for routine oral prophylaxis and may also be used in specialty offices for other recall treatment.
  CAT: Office Operations

113. Which of the following statements should be reworded on a patient's record to avoid litigation?
  c. This statement is insensitive to the patient's reactions and could be an issue in any potential litigation.
  CAT: Office Operations

114. What are the consequences of using a nickname or an incorrect name when filing an insurance claim form?
  b. If an insurance company does not have the accurate name of a patient, it will take longer to process a claim.
  CAT: Office Operations

115. Which of the following instruments is used to remove a tooth in one piece with the crown and root intact?
  b. A forceps is used to remove a tooth intact. A periosteal elevator is a surgical instrument used to separate the periosteum from bone. A surgical curette instrument is shaped like a scoop or spoon and is used to remove tissue. A rongeur is an instrument used to remove small, rough portions of bone.
  CAT: Chairside Dental Procedures

116. Which of the following burs is used to reduce the subgingival margin of a tooth during crown preparation?
  a. Flame diamond is used to reduce subgingival margins. A finishing bur is used to finish a restoration. A round bur and inverted cone are used during cavity preparation.
  CAT: Chairside Dental Procedures

117. The leading cause of tooth loss in adults is:
  c. Periodontal disease is the leading cause of tooth loss in adults. Almost 75% of American adults have some form of periodontal disease.
  CAT: Patient Education and Oral Health Management

118. The first step in patient education is to:
  c. Before beginning patient education, the dental health care professional should listen carefully to the patient to determine the patient's needs and to determine the patient's understanding of his or her dental health care.
  CAT: Patient Education and Oral Health Management

119. What would be a good source of protein for a person who eats a vegan diet?
  c. Legumes, such as beans, are seeds from a pod that are an excellent source of protein for a vegan diet. A vegan diet excludes eggs and steak. Carrots are not a source of protein.
  CAT: Patient Education and Oral Health Management

120. Which of the following topical anesthetics is the most widely used topical agent in dentistry?
  b. Benzocaine is a topical anesthesia. Articaine, bupivacaine, and levobupivacaine are local injection anesthesia.
  CAT: Chairside Dental Procedure

Radiation Health and Safety

1. Which of the following statements relates to working with a special needs patient?
   b. Always speak directly to a special needs patient. Offering assistance to a special needs patient displays caring, and the patient should be asked a question first before seeking input from the caregiver.
   CAT: Expose and Evaluate: Patient Management

2. Which of the following is a result of incorrect position-indicating device (PID) positioning?
   c. A herringbone pattern is created when the wrong side of the dental film is placed against the tooth or tissue surface to be examined. Missing a proximal surface is due to film placement, not beam placement. Overlap will occur if the beam is not properly aligned to the target area.
   CAT: Expose and Evaluate: Evaluate

3. What is the remedy to prevent overlapped contact areas on a radiographic image?
   d. Incorrect horizontal angulation results in overlapped contact areas. With correct horizontal angulation, the central ray is directed perpendicular to the curvature of the arch and through the contact areas of the teeth.
   CAT: Expose and Evaluate: Evaluate

4. What technique error will always be present on an occlusal radiograph using size 4 film?
   a. Size 4 film is larger than the end of the position-indicating device and will therefore always demonstrate a cone cut. The occlusal film is the largest intraoral film available, almost four times the size of a size 2 film. The other answers would not create a clear image like a cone cut.
   CAT: Expose and Evaluate: Evaluate

5. What is the function of intensifying screens used in extraoral radiography?
   d. The radiation dose from a panoramic radiograph is reduced by using intensifying screens in the cassettes. Intensifying screens are recommended because of less exposure of the patient to radiation.
   CAT: Radiation Safety for Patients and Operators

6. What is the term used to describe the area of ideal focus on a panoramic machine?
   b. The focal trough is the image layer of a panoramic machine; structures in the middle will be sharply depicted. The focal trough is the concept used to determine where the dental arches must be positioned to obtain the clearest image.
   CAT: Expose and Evaluate: Acquire

7. Which statement is true regarding the production of ghost images?
   d. Any removable metal object must be removed before panoramic exposure; failure to do so will result in a ghost image. Ghost images appear on the opposite side, somewhat higher, and are caused by metal objects.
   CAT: Expose and Evaluate: Evaluate

8. What type of radiograph should be prescribed when interproximal dental caries are suspected?
   b. Interproximal caries are best seen on bite-wing radiographs. The bite-wing image provides diagnostic information that cannot be obtained from any other source. An occlusal examination is a type of intraoral radiographic examination used to inspect all areas of the maxilla or the mandible in one image. A periapical is a radiographic examination that examines the tissues around the apex of the tooth. A panoramic is an extraoral image used to examine the upper and lower jaws on a single projection.
   CAT: Expose and Evaluate: Assessment and Preparation

9. What type of image shows the entire tooth, including the apex and surrounding structures?
   d. Periapical images reveal all of the crown and root, including the apex, alveolar crest, contact area, and surrounding bone. "Peri" refers to "around," and "apical" refers to the "apex of a tooth." An occlusal examination is a type of intraoral radiographic examination used to inspect all areas of the maxilla or the mandible in one image.
   CAT: Expose and Evaluate: Acquire

10. What is the proper technique to expose a bite-wing radiograph on a patient with mandibular tori?
   c. The receptor must be placed between the tori and the tongue and then exposed. When using the bite-wing technique, mandibular tori may cause problems with receptor placement and a modification in technique is necessary.
   CAT: Expose and Evaluate: Acquire

11. A size 1 intraoral receptor used on an adult patient would most likely image what area?
   b. Size 1 receptors are used for anterior views on adults and children. Size 1 receptors accommodate the mouths of most adults in the anterior regions. A full-mouth series of x-rays for an adult would usually involve receptor sizes 1 and 2. For adult bite-wing examinations, size 2 receptors are generally used.
   CAT: Expose and Evaluate: Assessment and Preparation

12. The following diagram depicts what type of radiographic exposure?
   d. The submentovertex is the radiographic exposure represented in the diagram. This is the under-the-chin exposure where the position-indicating device is under the patient's chin and the receptor is placed at the top of the patient's head at a right angle to the central ray. The other answers are extraoral exposures but not visible here.
   CAT: Expose and Evaluate: Acquire

13. What effect will occur by increasing the kilovoltage peak setting on the exposure control panel?
   b. A higher kilovoltage peak setting will produce more penetrating dental x-rays with greater energy and shorter wavelengths.
   CAT: Radiation Safety for Patients and Operators

14. Why is insulating oil added to the metal housing of the x-ray tubehead?
   b. The glass tube is immersed in oil to help absorb the heat created by x-ray production. Insulating oil prevents overheating by absorbing the heat created by the production of x-rays.
   CAT: Radiation Safety for Patients and Operators

15. The sharpness of a radiographic image is influenced by all of the following factors EXCEPT one. Which is the EXCEPTION?
   d. Sharpness is affected by the focal spot size, the composition of the image, and movement. The exception in this question is target-to-film distance.
   CAT: Expose and Evaluate: Evaluate

16. What type of radiograph is preferred to evaluate for a mandibular jaw fracture?
   d. The panoramic image is recommended for the evaluation of mandibular jaw fractures. On a panoramic image, a mandibular fracture appears as a radiolucent line at the site where the bone has separated.
   CAT: Expose and Evaluate: Assessment and Preparation

17. In which situation would extraoral radiography NOT be used?
   c. Extraoral radiography is not the best choice for diagnosis of dental caries. Bite-wing radiographs are used for this procedure.
   CAT: Expose and Evaluate: Assessment and Preparation

18. When exposing a molar bite-wing, the following conditions should exist EXCEPT:
   c. The anterior edge of the receptor should be placed at the midline of the mandibular second premolar to ensure that all the molars will be present in the molar bite-wing image.
   CAT: Expose and Evaluate: Acquire

19. An anterior periapical receptor is oriented _____, and a posterior periapical receptor is oriented _____:
   a. To ensure that all the apical regions and the entire tooth are visible on a periapical image, the receptor is placed vertically for an anterior periapical image and horizontally for a posterior periapical image.
   CAT: Expose and Evaluate: Acquire

20. Which rule governs the orientation of structures portrayed in two radiographs exposed at different angulations?
    b. The buccal object rule governs the orientation of structures portrayed in two radiographs exposed at different angulations. The buccal object rule can be used to determine the position of a root canal when there are multiple canals or to identify the position of a canal filled with gutta-percha in a maxillary tooth with two or more roots.
    CAT: Expose and Evaluate: Acquire

21. What piece of equipment is required to hold the receptor parallel to the long axis of the tooth in the paralleling technique?
    b. When using the paralleling technique, it is necessary to use some type of receptor holder. A variety of receptor holders are available, some designed for one-time use and others that can be sterilized.
    CAT: Expose and Evaluate: Assessment and Preparation

22. All of the following statements regarding duplicating film are true except one. What is the EXCEPTION?
    b. Duplicating film has emulsion on one side only. Duplicating film is sensitive to light, all procedures must be performed under darkroom conditions, and a duplicating machine is needed to produce the duplicate radiograph.
    CAT: Expose and Evaluate: Assessment and Preparation

23. Which of the following is NOT considered a critical organ with regards to dental radiography?
    c. The pituitary gland is not considered a critical organ and does not appear in the list of critical organs when the paralleling technique is used. The other organs are considered critical organs.
    CAT: Radiation Safety for Patients and Operators

24. When is a lead apron used?
    d. Proper patient protection when exposing any type or amount of radiographs is to protect patients by draping their bodies in a lead apron. Proper placement of the lead apron is from the neck over the shoulders and extending onto the lap. Make sure the patient's arms are tucked in the lead apron.
    CAT: Radiation Safety for Patients and Operators

25. A 5-year-old child fell while playing and needs a periapical radiograph of the anterior region of her maxilla. The child is very upset and uncooperative in the chair. Which of the following is the appropriate action?
    e. If the child is being uncooperative but a radiograph is required for proper treatment and diagnosis, the child should be placed on a parent's lap for comfort but both individuals need to be covered completely by the lead apron for proper protection of the critical organs and blood-forming tissues. The patient is exposed once to radiation whereas if a dental auxiliary held the film, she or he would be exposed multiple times.
    CAT: Expose and Evaluate: Patient Management

26. What does ALARA stand for?
    b. As low as reasonably achievable is the ultimate goal of any radiographer. We want to expose the patient to the least amount of radiation possible.
    CAT: Radiation Safety for Patients and Operators

27. Which of the following applies to producing radiographs on pregnant patients?
    c. American Dental Association (ADA) guidelines on producing radiographs are not altered for pregnant patients. The use of a lead apron is enough protection for the developing fetus or embryo.
    CAT: Radiation Safety for Patients and Operators

28. What is the maximum permissible dose a nonoccupationally exposed individual is allowed to accumulate in a year?
    b. The maximum dose equivalent that a body is permitted to receive in a specific period of time (nonoccupationally exposed) is 0.1 rem/year.
    CAT: Radiation Safety for Patients and Operators

29. What is the single best way to protect a patient from unnecessary radiation exposure?
    b. Fast film speed is the single most effective method of reducing a patient's exposure to radiation.
    CAT: Radiation Safety for Patients and Operators

30. Which collimator and PID reduce the amount of exposure a patient receives?
    d. Rectangular and 16-inch position-indicating devices (PIDs) are preferred because they produce less divergence of the x-ray beam. The rectangular lead collimator produces less of a target area outside of the film.
    CAT: Radiation Safety for Patients and Operators

31. Equipment filtration is comprised of which of the following?
    1. Inherent filtration
    2. Added filtration
    3. Total filtration
    a. Inherent filtration takes place when the primary beam passes through the unleaded glass window, the insulating oil, and the tubehead seal. It does not meet the standards regulated by state and federal law, so additional filtration is required. Added filtration is when the aluminum disc is placed between the collimator and the tubehead seal to filter out longer wavelength, lower energy x-rays from the x-ray beam. Total filtration is the sum of inherent and added filtration. Total filtration meets the regulations by state and federal law.
    CAT: Radiation Safety for Patients and Operators

32. What is the role of a collimator?
    c. The collimator is designed to restrict the size and shape of the x-ray beam, thus reducing the patient's exposure.
    CAT: Radiation Safety for Patients and Operators

33. How are film-holding devices used to protect the patient from exposure?
    a. Film-holding devices stabilize the film position in the mouth and reduce the chance for movement, thus ensuring that the "as low as reasonably achievable"

(ALARA) concept is being upheld by limiting retakes.
    CAT: Radiation Safety for Patients and Operators

34. Which of the following is true about the exposure of radiation on the body?
    a. Exposure to radiation can bring about changes in the individual's body chemicals, cells, tissues, and organs. The effects of radiation may not be determined for years.
    CAT: Radiation Safety for Patients and Operators

35. Which source produces the most annual radiation exposure to persons in the United States?
    a. Radon produces the most annual radiation exposure to persons in the United States. The majority of naturally occurring radiation is in the form of radon in the air.
    CAT: Radiation Safety for Patients and Operators

36. The following diagram depicts the correct positioning of the PID (position-indicating device) _____.
    b. The diagram represents positioning of the PID to prevent overlap, which is a horizontal angulation issue. The other answers do not refer to position of the PID for horizontal angulation using the cone shown.
    CAT: Radiation Safety for Patients and Operators

37. What is the size of the x-ray beam produced by a circular collimator as it reaches the patient's face?
    c. The x-ray beam produced by a circular collimator is 2.75 inches in diameter. A rectangular-shaped cone further reduces patient exposure to radiation as it is only slightly larger than size 2 intraoral film.
    CAT: Radiation Safety for Patients and Operators

38. Which PID would provide the most protection against radiation exposure for the patient?
    d. The patient is exposed to less radiation when a lead-lined, rectangular collimator is used.
    CAT: Radiation Safety for Patients and Operators

39. What is the purpose of including aluminum filtration inside the dental tubehead?
    c. The filter removes low energy x-rays from the beam, which adds to the absorbed dose for the patient. The aluminum discs filter out the longer wavelength, lower energy waves from the x-ray beam.
    CAT: Radiation Safety for Patients and Operators

40. Which of the following would be considered a short-term effect of radiation exposure?
    a. Short-term effects from radiation usually result from high doses; symptoms may include nausea. Genetic defects, cancer induction, and birth abnormalities would all be considered long-term effects of radiation exposure.
    CAT: Radiation Safety for Patients and Operators

41. What is the term to describe the time between radiation exposure and the appearance of the first clinical signs?
    a. The latent period is the time between exposure to radiation and the signs and symptoms of biologic damage. The observable effects of radiation are not visible immediately after exposure.
    CAT: Radiation Safety for Patients and Operators

42. Which cell would be considered radio-resistant?
    b. Muscle and nerve are among the most radio-resistant cells. These cells are radio-resistant because of their low mitotic activity and metabolism. Skin, oral mucosa, and reproductive cells are radio-sensitive cells.
    CAT: Radiation Safety for Patients and Operators

43. When the dental operator is producing a radiographic image on a patient, it is recommended that he or she stand at least how far away from the primary beam?
    d. Radiation health and safety guidelines require that the dental professional exposing a radiograph on a patient must stand 6 feet at a diagonal or perpendicular distance to ensure beam avoidance.
    CAT: Radiation Safety for Patients and Operators

44. What is the maximum permissible dose an occupationally exposed radiographer is allowed to accumulate in a year?
    a. The maximum dose equivalent that a body is permitted to receive in a specific period of time (occupationally exposed) is 5.0 rem/year.
    CAT: Radiation Safety for Patients and Operators

45. What can a radiographer wear to measure the daily amount of radiation exposure?
    c. A dosimeter badge is used to measure the amount of radiation an operator is being exposed to occupationally.
    CAT: Radiation Safety for Patients and Operators

46. Of the three forms of radiation, which is most detrimental to the patient and operator?
    d. X-radiation is comprised of primary, secondary, and scatter radiation. Primary radiation is composed of the x-ray beam that comes from the x-ray tube. Secondary radiation is when the source of radiation interacts with matter. Scatter radiation is when the radiation is deflected from its path. Thus scatter radiation is the most detrimental to the operator and patient.
    CAT: Radiation Safety for Patients and Operators

47. Why is it important for a radiographer to understand ionizing radiation?
    c. Ionizing radiation causes harmful effects to humans and their cellular metabolism and permanent damage to living cells and tissues.
    CAT: Radiation Safety for Patients and Operators

48. What is the best way for the dental operator to prevent exposure to x-radiation?
    a. The dental radiographer must use proper protection measures to prevent occupational exposure to x-radiation; guidelines are based upon the rule "the dental radiographer must avoid the primary beam."
    CAT: Radiation Safety for Patients and Operators

49. Which of the following statements relates to working with a patient with a physical challenge or one with special needs?
    b. Always speak directly to a patient with a disability. Offering assistance to a patient with a disability displays caring, and the patient should be asked questions first before input from the caregiver is sought.
    CAT: Expose and Evaluate: Patient Management

50. Which of the following is an advantage of digital radiography?
    b. Digital radiography has several advantages over film. Primarily, it eliminates the need for x-ray film, processing solutions, running water, and a darkroom and can eliminate potential processing errors. Digital radiography does not eliminate the potential of exposure errors, however.
    CAT: Expose and Evaluate: Assessment and Preparation

51. What technique should the dental assistant use on a patient with a gag reflex?
    b. To prevent the patient from gagging, it is necessary to avoid any tactile stimuli to the gag reflex area.
    CAT: Expose and Evaluate: Patient Management

52. What is the traditional statute of limitations for adult radiographs?
    b. Although some states have specific guidelines for maintaining radiographs, 7 years is the traditional statute of limitations.
    CAT: Radiology Regulations

53. Which device is used to restrict the size and shape of the x-ray beam and to reduce patient exposure?
    c. Collimation is used to restrict the size and shape of the x-ray beam and to reduce patient exposure. A collimator, or lead plate with a hole in the middle, is fitted directly over the opening of the machine housing where the x-ray beam exits the tubehead.
    CAT: Quality Assurance

54. What is the purpose of a dosimeter?
    c. A dosimeter is worn by the x-ray operator to measure any radiation exposure over a set period of time. If the operator follows all safety measures, the processed dosimeter should read zero.
    CAT: Radiation Safety for Patients and Operators

55. Commercially available barrier envelopes _____.
    b. Barrier envelopes that fit over intraoral films can be used to protect the film packets from saliva and minimize contamination after exposure of the film.
    CAT: Infection Control: Standard Precautions for Equipment

56. Which type of PID would be most effective in reducing patient exposure?
    d. The 16-inch rectangular PID provides the most effective reduction of x-radiation during routine patient exposures.
    CAT: CAT: Radiology Regulations

57. The time interval between radiographic examinations for children should be _____.
    d. As with all patients, the time interval and the number of radiographs prescribed for children should be based on the individual needs of the child.
    CAT: Radiation Safety for Patients and Operators

58. Which of the following is the greatest source of cross-contamination in dental radiology?
    b. The film packet is potentially the greatest source for cross-contamination in dental radiology; improper handling of the film creates contamination issues in the operatory and in the darkroom. Gloves prevent cross-contamination; the lead apron is disinfected after every patient; and the beam alignment device is sterilized after each patient.
    CAT: Infection Control: Standard Precautions for Equipment

59. Which of the following is a result of improper storage of x-ray film?
    a. Grayish film may result if the film is stored in hot or cold areas or stored in an area with chemicals. A clear film is the result

of too long in the fixer or no exposure to radiation, whereas a black film is the result of exposure to white light. A white film is a misnomer as white refers to radiopaque, which is not related to storage issues.
CAT: Quality Assurance

60. Which of the following is recommended by the CDC?

    d. Because cross contamination is very possible, the Centers for Disease Control and Prevention (CDC) recommends proper personal protective equipment (PPE) for the operator including a mask and eyewear. Placing films in harsh solutions may damage the emulsion in the film packet and necessitate a retake; an intermediate-level Environmental Protection Agency (EPA)-registered disinfectant should be used, and a semicritical item must be heat sterilized.
    CAT: Infection Control: Standard Precautions for Patient and Operators

61. Which of the following components of the tubehead protects the patient by removing long-wave energy?

    b. The filter protects the patient by removing the long wave energy that is harmful to the tissue from the primary beam. The window is a component of the tubehead designed to allow x-ray energy to pass through it to the patient and is not a patient protection. The lead-lined PID protects the patient by restricting the size of the primary beam, and the collimator protects the patient by limiting the size of the primary beam to 2¾ inches from the patient's face.
    CAT: CAT: Radiology Regulations

62. Which of the following would be helpful to a patient who is uncertain about having dental radiographs taken?

    d. An educated response to electing a dental procedure is always the best option, for both patient and dental professional. It would be helpful to determine whether the patient has a gag reflex that might be triggered by an intraoral procedure, and information regarding insurance benefits

is likewise useful. But the education the patient needs in order to make an informed decision is on the value of dental radiographs in diagnosis (or problems with diagnosis), many times providing a measure of protection.
CAT: Expose and Evaluate: Patient Management

63. One of the greatest services a dental professional can provide for patients is a: _____.

    b. Providing services for a patient via an appropriate oral examination and dental radiographs is of course a benefit. Likewise, taking a thorough medical and dental history is a professional responsibility. The best service with long-term effect is providing the patient with comprehensive dental health education.
    CAT: Expose and Evaluate: Patient Management

64. Packaged dental radiography film is affected by all except:_____.

    d. Light, humidity, and radiation affect stored dental film; ultraviolet light does not.
    CAT: Quality Assurance

65. Which of the following describes the frequency with which processing solutions must be changed?

    a. Processing solutions need to be replaced as chemicals begin to become depleted, approximately every 3-4 weeks of use.
    CAT: Quality Assurance

66. A yellow-brown color on a developed film would indicate which of the following?

    b. Exhausted fixer causes yellowing of the dental image; exhausted developer causes a light image; a dirty processing tank will cause dark spots; a warm temperature will cause a dark image.
    CAT: Quality Assurance

67. The optimal storage temperature for dental film is: _____.

    b. Dental film should not be stored below 50 degrees F or above 70 degrees F.
    CAT: Quality Assurance

68. When stocking dental radiographic film, it is best to apply which of the following rules of thumb?

    a. A good rule of thumb when storing and using dental x-ray film is last in (the film with the furthest from the current day's date) first out (the films should be used first, prior to other films).

    CAT: Quality Assurance

69. When intensifying screens are not in perfect contact with the screen film, which of the following will result?

    c. When intensifying screens are not in perfect contact with the screen film, the film quality will be disturbed. The image will not be as clear or as sharp when there is a separation of screen and film. The separation will not damage the film or screen, and the image will not darken.

    CAT: Quality Assurance

70. Sodium sulfite in the developer solution is responsible for_____.

    b. Sodium sulfite in the developer is responsible for preventing rapid oxidation. Hydroquinone converts exposed silver halide crystals to dark metallic silver. Sodium carbonate activates the developer agents. Sodium carbonate softens the gelatin of the film emulsion.

    CAT: Quality Assurance

71. Creating an identical copy of a set of radiographs is called _____.

    a. Creating an identical copy of a set of radiographs is called film duplication.

    CAT: Radiology Regulations

72. Uses of duplicate films include all EXCEPT _____.

    b. Duplicate dental images are used for insurance purposes, referral to a specialist, and for teaching. They are not used to create a copy for a patient's personal use.

    CAT: Radiology Regulations

73. The improper exposure of a dental radiograph may result in which of the following?

    b. Improper x-ray exposure can result in a malpractice lawsuit but would not be considered insurance fraud. A phobia is an irrational fear; functioning under a standard of care would prevent an improper exposure.

    CAT: Radiology Regulations

74. Informed consent implies that the patient has received _____.

    c. To be fully informed in order to consent to a procedure, full disclosure is required.

    CAT: Radiology Regulations

75. The dental record is a legal document.

    a. True. The dental record is a legal record and should only be written on in ink or via data recorded on a computer.

    CAT: Radiology Regulations

76. Which of the following is the final step in film duplication?

    a. The steps in film duplication would include: arranging the radiographs on the light source, placing the duplicating film on the arranged radiographs, securing the lid, and setting the timer. The final step is labeling the radiographic mount.

    CAT: Radiology Regulations

77. The longer duplicating film is exposed to light, _____.

    c. The lightness of a duplicated film is directly proportional to the amount of time it is exposed to light. The longer the exposure, the lighter the film.

    CAT: Radiology Regulations

78. A blurred image on a duplication film is likely caused by which of the following?

    b. Blurred duplicate images are caused by poor contact between the source film and the duplicating film. Film quality, unless expired, is not a cause, and even then it would not result in a blurred image. Incorrect exposure times will result in light or dark films, not blurred.

    CAT: Radiology Regulations

79. Used developer solution must be disposed of in which of the following ways?

    b. Used developer is considered nonhazardous waste and can be disposed of in the sanitary drain.

    CAT: Radiology Regulations

80. Which of the following infection control protocols applies to radiography procedures?
  a. Standard Precautions apply to all dental procedures.
    CAT: Infection Control: Standard Precautions for Equipment

81. Dental x-ray equipment is classified as _____.
  d. Dental x-ray equipment is classified as semi- and noncritical instruments because it contacts but does not penetrate soft tissue or bone and/or does not contact mucous membranes. No critical instruments (those used to penetrate soft tissue or bone) are used in dental radiography.
    CAT: Infection Control: Standard Precautions for Equipment

82. Prior to dental film exposure, which of the following must be covered or disinfected?
  a. The x-ray machine needs to be covered or disinfected prior to use. The towel dispenser is out of the field of contamination, and the beam alignment device and image receptors are sterile.
    CAT: Infection Control: Standard Precautions for Equipment

83. Which is a correct statement concerning disinfection procedures for the darkroom?
  a. In the darkroom, countertops and areas touched with gloved hands need to be disinfected.
    CAT: Infection Control: Standard Precautions for Equipment

84. EPA-registered chemical germicides labeled as a *tuberculocidal* are classified as _____.
  b. EPA-registered chemical germicides labeled as *tuberculocidal* are classified as intermediate-level disinfectants. EPA-registered chemical germicides labeled as *hospital disinfectants* are classified as low-level disinfectants. EPA-registered chemical germicides labeled as *sterilants* are classified as high-level disinfectants.
    CAT: Infection Control: Standard Precautions for Equipment

85. Films removed from barrier envelopes are processed with _____.
  b. Dental films that have been protected by a barrier covering can be processed, once the barrier is removed, by an ungloved hand.
    CAT: Infection Control: Standard Precautions for Equipment

86. Beam alignment devices must be _____.
  a. Beam alignment devices must be sterilized. Disinfection or decontamination processes are not adequate infection control measures.
    CAT: Infection Control: Standard Precautions for Equipment

87. The three types of hand hygiene advised for radiography procedures include all EXCEPT which of the following?
  b. The three types of hand hygiene advised for radiographic procedures are a routine handwashing, antiseptic handwashing, and antiseptic hand rub. Aseptic handwashing is required for more invasive procedures, such as surgery.
    CAT: Infection Control: Standard Precautions for Patient and Operators

88. A needle-stick injury would result in which type of exposure to infectious disease?
  b. Parenteral exposure is exposure to blood or other infectious materials that results from piercing or puncturing the skin barrier, such as a needle-stick injury. An occupational exposure defines the types of risks one might expect from a given occupation; the terms *critical* and *semicritical* apply to categories of instruments.
    CAT: Infection Control: Standard Precautions for Patient and Operators

89. An instrument used to penetrate soft tissue or bone is considered a _____ instrument.
  a. An instrument that contacts mucous membranes and penetrates soft tissue or bone is considered a critical instrument. An instrument that does not contact mucous membranes is considered a noncritical instrument. An instrument that

contacts mucous membranes but does not penetrate soft tissue or bone is considered a semicritical instrument.

CAT: Infection Control: Standard Precautions for Patient and Operators

90. Which statement is correct concerning the use of gloves during a radiography procedure?

c. Fresh gloves need to be worn for each new patient. Washing them with soap and water or chemicals would decrease their barrier-protection properties.

CAT: Infection Control: Standard Precautions for Patient and Operators

91. Which of the following statements is correct regarding the use of masks and protective eyewear during radiographic procedures?

c. Due to the minimal risk of splash or spatter in a radiography procedure, the use of a face mask and protective eyewear are optional.

CAT: Infection Control: Standard Precautions for Patient and Operators

92. At the end of the radiography procedure, the operator should remove the lead apron from the patient with hands that are _____.

b. The operator should remove the lead apron from the patient at the end of the procedure with ungloved hands.

CAT: Infection Control: Standard Precautions for Patient and Operators

93. Dental films contaminated with saliva should be _____.

b. Dental films contaminated with saliva should be placed in a cup labeled with the patient's name.

CAT: Infection Control: Standard Precautions for Patient and Operators

94. Infection control procedures in dental radiography can be divided into which segments/categories?

a. The four infection control processes involved in dental radiography occur

before exposure, during exposure, after exposure, and in processing.

CAT: Infection Control: Standard Precautions for Patient and Operators

95. The protocol that protects patients from cross-contamination in a radiographic procedures is _____.

a. Standard Precautions protect both the patient and dental healthcare worker from cross-contamination.

CAT: Infection Control: Standard Precautions for Patient and Operators

96. Bite guides of the panoramic or cephalometric x-ray machine should be _____.

e. Bite guides should be sterilized and disinfected. They are not single-use items

CAT: Infection Control: Standard Precautions for Patient and Operators

97. Beam alignment devices can be placed on _____.

e. A beam alignment device can be place on a disinfected, covered surface.

CAT: Infection Control: Standard Precautions for Patient and Operators

98. The operator should clean and disinfect any uncovered areas while wearing _____.

c. Vinyl, latex, and powderless gloves are inadequate protection during the use of a disinfectant. Utility gloves must be worn during disinfection procedures.

CAT: Infection Control: Standard Precautions for Patient and Operators

99. To what radiopaque landmark are the arrows pointing?

a. The mental ridge is the radiopaque landmark indicated by the arrows in this mandibular central incisor projection. Torus mandibularis appears as rounded, dense radiopaque bone. Genial tubercles are seen in this projection, but they are the radiopaque "donut" surrounding the lingual foramen below the apices of the central incisors. The mylohyoid ridge is seen only on the mandibular molar projection.

CAT: **Expose and Evaluate: Evaluate**

100. This radiograph is an example of which processing error?

    a. The radiograph is an example of reticulation, or cracked emulsion, which is

a result of drastic temperature differences between the developing solution and water tank. Fixer spots are uneven white spots; developer spots would be dark spots; and air bubbles are small, circular white spots.

CAT: **Expose and Evaluate: Evaluate**

Infection Control

1. After accepting employment you opt not to receive a hepatitis B vaccination and have signed a waiver to this effect, you have the right to:

    b. In accordance with the OSHA Bloodborne Pathogens Standard, an employee who initially declines the vaccination may at a later date, while still covered under the standard, decide to accept the offer. The employer must make the vaccine available at no charge at that time.

    CAT: **Patient and Dental Healthcare Worker Education**

2. All dental professionals must use surgical masks and protective eyewear to protect the eyes and face:

    c. In accordance with OSHA recommendations, surgical masks and protective eyewear are to be worn whenever splashes, spray, spatter, or droplets of blood or saliva may be generated and eye, nose, or mouth contamination may occur.

    CAT: **Preventing Cross-Contamination and Disease Transmission**

3. All dental assistants involved in direct patient care must undergo routine training in:

    a. The OSHA standard requires that employers must ensure that all employees with occupational exposure participate in a training program on the hazards associated with body fluids, safety issues, hazard communication, and the protective techniques needed to be taken to minimize the risk of occupational exposure.

    CAT: **Occupational Safety**

4. When immunity is present at birth, it is referred to as:

    d. When immunity is present at birth, it is called inherited immunity. Immunity that is developed during a person's lifetime is called acquired immunity.

    CAT: **Patient and Dental Healthcare Worker Education**

5. _____ immunity occurs when a vaccination is administered and the body forms antibodies in response to the vaccine.

    b. When a human body has not been exposed to a disease, it has not developed antibodies and is completely defenseless against the disease. Antibodies can be introduced into the body artificially by immunization or vaccination. The body then forms antibodies in response to the vaccine; this is known as active artificial immunity.

    CAT: **Patient and Dental Healthcare Worker Education**

6. A chronic infection is best exemplified by which of the following?

    a. A chronic infection is one of long duration.

    CAT: **Patient and Dental Healthcare Worker Education**

7. Which of the following exemplifies an acute infection?

    c. An acute infection is of short duration but may be severe.

    CAT: **Patient and Dental Healthcare Worker Education**

8. Microorganisms that produce disease in humans are known as:
   b. A pathogen is a microorganism or substance capable of producing a disease.
   CAT: Patient and Dental Healthcare Worker Education

9. Bacteria can be identified by shape. Which of the following is the shape of bacilli?
   b. Bacteria can be found in only three shapes: spherical, rod, or spiral. Bacilli are rods, cocci are spherical, and spirochetes are spiral.
   CAT: Patient and Dental Healthcare Worker Education

10. An infection that results from a defective immune system that cannot defend against pathogens normally found in the environment is a(n):
    d. An opportunistic infection results from a defective immune system that cannot defend against pathogens normally found in the environment. These infections are seen in patients receiving large doses of steroids or other immunosuppressive drugs and in patients with acquired immunodeficiency syndrome.
    CAT: Patient and Dental Healthcare Worker Education

11. Which of the following is an example of parenteral disease transmission in dentistry?
    d. Parenteral disease transmission can occur with a needle stick injury, human bites, cuts, abrasions, or any break in the skin. The other answers refer to direct, indirect, and droplet forms of transmission.
    CAT: Preventing Cross-Contamination and Disease Transmission

12. The transmission of a disease to a susceptible person by handling contaminated instruments or by touching the face, eyes, or mouth is referred to as:
    c. The indirect transfer of organisms to a susceptible person can occur by handling contaminated instruments or touching contaminated surfaces and then touching the face, eyes, or mouth.
    CAT: Preventing Cross-Contamination and Disease Transmission

13. Which of the following would be considered the best method for determining whether there is proper sterilization function of a sterilizer?
    c. Biologic monitoring, or spore testing, is the only way to determine if sterilization has occurred and all bacteria and endospores have been killed. The CDC, ADA, and OSAP all recommend at least weekly biologic monitoring of sterilization equipment.
    CAT: Instrument Processing

14. When a package of hazardous infectious waste is being prepared for disposal, which of the following should be considered?
    a. When waste leaves the office, the EPA regulations apply to the disposal. All waste containers that hold potentially infectious materials, whether regulated or nonregulated, must be placed in closable, leak-proof containers or bags that are color coded or labeled appropriately with the biohazard symbol.
    CAT: Instrument Processing

15. Which of the following PPE is removed first after the completion of a clinical procedure?
    c. The gown is removed first by reaching back and pulling it over the gloves and turning it inside out.
    CAT: Preventing Cross-Contamination and Disease Transmission

16. Exam gloves used during dental treatment can be made of:
    a. Gloves used during routine examination and treatment may be made of vinyl, latex, or nitrile. Thin plastic may serve as an overglove, dermal cloth gloves may be used to handle heated items, and heavy nitrile gloves are used in preparing instruments for sterilization.
    CAT: Preventing Cross-Contamination and Disease Transmission

17. Which of the following is considered regulated waste (biohazard)?
    b. Regulated waste is contaminated waste that is capable of transmitting an infectious disease. Pathologic waste, such as soft tissue and extracted teeth, are regulated waste.

Paper from mixing pads may go into general waste. Spent fixer is a hazardous waste, and barriers used during treatment typically are not considered infectious waste unless for some reason they become blood soaked.
CAT: Occupational Safety

18. Which of the following statements is true as it applies to the use of overgloves?
    b. Overgloves are used only as an alternative to changing gloves in situations when the assistant may need to leave the chair to obtain a material or enter a cabinet drawer and want to prevent contaminating an area without changing gloves. They are made of thin plastic and do not come in contact with the skin.
    CAT: Preventing Cross-Contamination and Disease Transmission

19. During which of the following procedures would you use sterile surgical gloves?
    b. During invasive procedures, such as surgery, it would be necessary to wear sterile surgical gloves.
    CAT: Occupational Safety

20. The most common route of disease transmission in the dental office is through:
    b. For the dental health team, the most common route of disease transmission is direct contact with the patient's blood or saliva.
    CAT: Preventing Cross-Contamination and Disease Transmission

21. The strength of an organism in its ability to produce disease is:
    a. After microorganisms enter the body, three basic factors determine whether an infectious disease will develop: virulence (the pathogenic properties of the invading microorganism), dose (the number of microorganisms that invade the body), and resistance (the body's defense mechanism of the host).
    CAT: Maintaining Aseptic Conditions

22. The use of a preprocedural mouth rinse can lower the number of microorganisms that may escape a patient's mouth through which of the following routes?
    a. The number of microorganisms is reduced in the aerosols, spray, and spatter

from the mouth. The indirect transfer of organisms to a susceptible person can occur by handling contaminated instruments or touching contaminated surfaces and then touching the face, eyes, or mouth. Oral mouthwash will not reduce microorganisms from this method of transmission.
CAT: Maintaining Aseptic Conditions

23. _____ infection is the mode of disease transmission that involves large-particle droplet spatter. ____ infection involves minute particles that can remain in the air for hours and can be inhaled.
    c. Whereas large particle spatter is referred to as droplet infection, the small particle size droplet can remain in the air for hours and is referred to as airborne infection.
    CAT: Maintaining Aseptic Conditions

24. Pathogens that are carried in the blood and body fluids of infected individuals and that can be transmitted to others are referred to as:
    a. Bloodborne pathogens are disease-producing microorganisms that are carried in the blood and body fluids of infected individuals and that can be transmitted to others.
    CAT: Occupational Safety

25. Recommendations concerning gloves would fall under which of the following categories of infection control practices that directly relate to dental radiography procedures?
    a. The wearing of gloves during patient treatment is a standard precaution and one of the pieces of personal protective equipment (PPE).
    CAT: Asepsis Procedures

26. Protective clothing:
    a. The OSHA standard requires that protective clothing such as laboratory coats and jackets must be worn to prevent skin mucous membrane exposure when contact with blood or other bodily fluids is anticipated.
    CAT: Preventing Cross-Contamination and Disease Transmission

27. When using medical latex or vinyl gloves, _____.
    b. Nonsterile gloves are recommended for examinations and nonsurgical procedures. Sterile gloves are worn during invasive surgical procedures.
    CAT: **Preventing Cross-Contamination and Disease Transmission**

28. _____ is defined as the absence of pathogens, or disease-causing microorganisms.
    d. The term *asepsis* refers to a "sterile state; a condition free from germs, infection and any form of life."
    CAT: **Asepsis Procedures**

29. Define antiseptic.
    b. *Antisepsis* means "anti" (against) + "sepsis" (putrefaction). This is the prevention of sepsis by preventing or inhibiting the growth of causative microorganisms. Thus, antiseptic is the substance that inhibits the growth of bacteria.
    CAT: **Asepsis Procedures**

30. While taking a patient's health history, it is noted that there is a history of tuberculosis and the patient is currently experiencing symptoms of this disease. Which of the following would *not* be appropriate action in the office?
    b. The patient should not be told you are unable to treat him or her. Rather, arrangements should be made to determine the state of the disease and then defer any elective treatment until the patient has been released by the physician. Emergency dental care can be provided in an isolation setting.
    CAT: **Patient and Dental Healthcare Worker Education**

31. When can a liquid sterilant or high-level disinfectant achieve sterilization?
    b. Sterilization will occur with a high-level disinfectant when the solution is used only for longer exposure times consistent with manufacturer's directions.
    CAT: **Instrument Processing**

32. Which of the following may be used for surface disinfectant in the dental office?
    a. From this list, the iodophors would be the best choice for a surface disinfectant.

    It is a well-known killing agent but does have some undesirable properties of corrosiveness, irritation of tissues, and allergenicity.
    CAT: **Instrument Processing**

33. Before dental x-ray films are exposed, the treatment area must be prepared using:
    b. As with all treatment, before the procedure, the treatment area must be prepared using aseptic techniques.
    CAT: **Asepsis Procedures**

34. Manufacturers of sterilizers (autoclaves) set them to reach a maximum steam temperature of ___°F and pressure of ___ pounds per square inch (psi).
    a. Most manufacturers preset the sterilizers to reach a maximum steam temperature of 250 to 260°F and a pressure of 15 to 30 psi.
    CAT: **Instrument Processing**

35. According to CDC guidelines, when transporting a biopsy specimen, it should be:
    b. According to CDC guidelines, when transporting a biopsy specimen, it should be placed in a sturdy, leak-proof container labeled with a biohazard symbol.
    CAT: **Occupational Safety**

36. Instruments must be absolutely dry or they will rust or have an ash layer when using which type of sterilization process?
    a. When using the chemical vapor processing method for sterilizing instruments, it is absolutely necessary to dry the instruments or they will rust or have an ash layer left on the surface.
    CAT: **Instrument Processing**

37. Which of the following are considered to be semi critical instruments in radiography?
    d. The CDC categorizes patient care items according to critical, semicritical, or noncritical based on the potential risk of infection during use of the items. An x-ray holding device is a semicritical item that is heat resistant and, at a minimum, must be cleaned and treated with a high-level disinfectant.
    CAT: **Asepsis Procedures**

38. Which of the following statements is true concerning cleaning and disinfection of the dental unit and environmental surfaces?
   a. The dental unit is subjected to aerosols and would be subjected to blood and saliva spatter; thus, the intermediate level of disinfection is necessary.
   CAT: **Asepsis Procedures**

39. Which method of sterilization requires good ventilation?
   c. The unsaturated chemical vapor system of sterilization requires good ventilation in the sterilization area because of possible vapors being released into the environment.
   CAT: **Maintaining Aseptic Conditions**

40. Which method is used to sterilize unwrapped instruments for immediate use?
   d. Flash sterilization is a method used to sterilize unwrapped patient care items for immediate use. The unwrapped instruments are no longer sterile after they are removed from the sterilizer.
   CAT: **Instrument Processing**

41. From the list below, select the best procedure for caring for an explorer.
   a. The sharp points on an explorer require that these tips be protected with an emulsion before steam under pressure sterilization.
   CAT: **Instrument Processing**

42. From the list below, select the best procedure for caring for a mouth mirror.
   b. Emulsion on a mirror will possibly leave a film on the mirror; thus, it can be sterilized under steam under pressure without an emulsion. The other two methods are not acceptable methods of sterilizing the mirror.
   CAT: **Instrument Processing**

43. From the list below, select the best procedure for caring for a pair of crown and collar scissors.
   a. The sharp edges on the beaks of the scissors require that these beaks be protected with an emulsion before steam-under-pressure sterilization.
   CAT: **Instrument Processing**

44. From the list below, select the best procedure for caring for a handpiece.
   b. Emulsion on a handpiece may conflict with the manufacturer's recommendations; thus, most handpieces can be sterilized by steam under pressure without an emulsion. In all cases, the manufacturer's directions should be consulted before sterilizing a handpiece for the first time.
   CAT: **Instrument Processing**

45. From the list below, select the best procedure for caring for a saliva ejector.
   d. Saliva ejectors are manufactured for one-time use only.
   CAT: **Instrument Processing**

46. From the list below, select the best procedure for caring for a contaminated needle.
   c. All needles are placed in a sharps container.
   CAT: **Preventing Cross-Contamination and Disease Transmission**

47. From the list below, select the best procedure for caring for a pair of protective glasses.
   c. CDC guidelines recommend that eyewear be cleaned with soap and water, or if the eyewear is visibly soiled, reusable facial protective wear can be cleaned and disinfected between patients.
   CAT: **Preventing Cross-Contamination and Disease Transmission**

48. From the list below, select the best procedure for caring for medication bottles.
   d. Medication bottles are reused at chairside and must be disinfected. This is best accomplished by spray–wipe–spray or wipe–wait–wipe. If using a spray, the first spray–wipe is to clean, and then the surface is sprayed a second time to disinfect, and it remains to dry. If using wipes, the first wipe is to clean, and the second wipe is to disinfect.
   CAT: **Asepsis Procedures**

49. Which type of sterilization used in the dental office requires the highest temperature?
   c. Dry heat sterilization requires the highest degree of heat and the longest time.
   CAT: **Instrument Processing**

50. Immersion in a chemical liquid sterilant requires at least ____ hour(s) of contact time for sterilization to occur.
   c. Immersion in a chemical liquid sterilant requires at least 10 hours of contact time for sterilization to occur, according to most manufacturers.
   CAT: Asepsis Procedures

51. Which of the following is *not* a recommended method for sterilizing dental burs?
   a. Burs are sterilized in steam under pressure. The other methods could damage burs, and flash sterilization is not an option because the bur would need to be used immediately to maintain sterility.
   CAT: Instrument Processing

52. Select the ideal instrument processing area.
   b. To avoid disease transmission, the instrument processing area or sterilization area should be within the dental suite and dedicated only to instrument processing. Excess size is not necessary because only the persons responsible for the sterilization process should be in the area.
   CAT: Instrument Processing

53. There are areas of the instrument processing facility that govern the workflow pattern. The processing should flow in a single loop from:
   b. In designing an instrument processing area, the facility should flow in a single loop from dirty to clean to sterile to storage. The other responses do not follow this sequence.
   CAT: Instrument Processing

54. What is the purpose of a holding solution?
   c. If instruments cannot be cleaned immediately after a procedure is performed, they may be placed in a holding (presoaking) solution. This process facilitates the cleaning process by preventing debris from drying on the instruments. It does not clean, disinfect, or sterilize the instruments.
   CAT: Asepsis Procedures

55. The least desirable method of precleaning dental instruments is:
   a. Hand washing must be avoided because it can potentially cause glove punctures

and result in injury to the assistant. The ulltrasonic cleaner and instrument washing machines both clean the instruments safely, but the holding solution does not clean the instruments.
   CAT: Instrument Processing

56. The ultrasonic cleaner should be cleaned and disinfected:
   c. Every day the ultrasonic cleaner should be cleaned and disinfected before using it the next day to provide a clean tank for processing the next day's instruments. The other answers are not appropriate times.
   CAT: Instrument Processing

57. After instruments have completed the cleaning cycle of the ultrasonic cleaner, they should be:
   b. Instruments are placed in the ultrasonic cleaner for the appropriate time and then rinsed thoroughly before the next steps in processing. Various steps are followed depending on the type of instrument, and only after the appropriate process are the instruments stored.
   CAT: Instrument Processing

58. The ultrasonic cleaner:
   a. The ultrasonic cleaner does only cleaning and removal of debris. It does not prewash, disinfect, or sterilize.
   CAT: Instrument Processing

59. Why is it important to keep an MSDS for the liquid sterilant (e.g., glutaraldehyde) on file?
   b. The MSDS provides valuable information on how to manage an exposure if one occurs. It does not relate to any records management procedures, and it will not prevent an exposure.
   CAT: Occupational Safety

60. The process that kills disease-causing microorganisms, but not necessarily all microbial life, is called:
   c. Disinfection is capable of destroying some microorganisms but not all microbial life. Therefore, when possible, all items that can be should be sterilized or discarded.

Precleaning or cleaning is the removal of bioburden before disinfection. Sterilization is the process that kills all microorganisms.
CAT: Asepsis Procedures

61. Spores of *Bacillus atrophaeus* are used to monitor which of the following types of sterilizers?
    b. Biologic indicators contain the bacterial endospores used for monitoring. The spores used are *Geobacillus stearothermophilus* for steam under pressure and *Bacillus atrophaeus* for dry heat.
    CAT: Instrument Processing

62. Patient care instruments are categorized into various classifications. Into which classification would instruments such as surgical forceps, scalpels, bone chisels, and scalers be placed?
    a. All of these instruments are in the critical category because they are used in invasive procedures and must be cleaned and sterilized by heat. Semicritical instruments, such as mouth mirrors and plastic instruments, touch mucous membranes but do not touch bone or penetrate soft tissue. Noncritical instruments, such as an x-ray head, only contact intact skin.
    CAT: Instrument Processing

63. For which of the following is there *not* a vaccine?
    d. Strep throat is a disease for which there is not a vaccine. For each of the other diseases, there is some form of vaccine.
    CAT: Patient and Dental Healthcare Worker Education

64. Select the heat sterilization method that requires good ventilation in the dental office.
    c. Chemical vapor sterilization is a method by means of hot formaldehyde vapors under pressure. The other methods do not use chemicals.
    CAT: Instrument Processing

65. *Legionella* bacteria can cause what type of condition in susceptible persons?
    b. This bacteria occurs naturally in water and may be resistant to some chlorines in domestic water because they can exist inside certain free-living amoebae as the causative agent of a type of pneumonia called Legionnaires disease. These bacteria do not impact the other organs.
    CAT: Patient and Dental Healthcare Worker Education

66. Nosocomial infections are commonly acquired in:
    c. Nosocomial infections are those infections commonly acquired in a hospital or other medical setting. They are not likely to be acquired in the other settings.
    CAT: Patient and Dental Healthcare Worker Education

67. According to OSHA, the dental assistant may do which of the following before depositing a contaminated needle in a designated puncture-resistant container?
    a. Needles are recapped in a recapping device at chairside after being used and then discarded in the sharps container. None of the other options are acceptable methods of handling a needle before placing it in a puncture-resistant container.
    CAT: Occupational Safety

68. OSHA requires a *minimum* period of training of dental personnel in which of the following areas?
    b. OSHA requires that employees receive training in the Bloodborne Pathogens Standard, the Hazard Communication Standard, and general safety standards. The other three standards do not exist.
    CAT: Occupational Safety

69. Which of the following is the goal of a sound infection control program to reduce cross-contamination?
    c. The goal of an infection control program seeks to reduce cross-contamination from dental team members to other patients. A sound infection control program also seeks to reduce cross-contamination not only from patient to patient and patient to dental team members, but there is no viable recognized program of the community to the dental practice.
    CAT: Patient and Dental Healthcare Worker Education.

70. Which of the following statements is true as it relates to the environmental infection control in a clinical area?
    b. Hard surfaces are much easier to maintain and do not collect debris and materials; thus, carpet and cloth–upholstered furnishings in the treatment area should be avoided.
    CAT: Asepsis Procedures

71. The Organization for Safety and Asepsis Procedures (OSAP) identifies the classification of clinical touch surfaces to include which of the following?
    b. OSAP identifies light handles, dental unit controls, and chair switches as clinical touch surfaces. Many touch surfaces are identified in the other answers, but there is a distracter in each of these other answers that makes them inaccurate.
    CAT: Occupational Safety

72. Which of the following is a recommended method of preventing surface contamination?
    a. The use of a surface barrier made of fluid–resistant material is recommended. The use of alcohol is not acceptable by any of the agencies that are concerned with dental office treatment areas. The other two answers are not necessary when the surface barrier is used unless there is spatter evident.
    CAT: Asepsis Procedures

73. What are standard precautions?
    c. Standard precautions, referred to in the OSHA Bloodborne Pathogens Standard, are based on the concept that all human blood and body fluids (including saliva) are to be treated as if known to be infected with bloodborne diseases.
    CAT: Occupational Safety

74. The best time to clean and disinfect a dental prosthesis or impression that will be processed in the office laboratory is:
    d. A prosthesis should be cleaned as soon as possible after removal from a patient's mouth to avoid potential cross-contamination and to avoid allowing the prosthesis to have time to dry out.
    CAT: Asepsis Procedures

75. A victim who immediately feels the effects of a chemical spill with symptoms of dizziness, headache, nausea, and vomiting, is experiencing:
    b. Acute chemical toxicity results from high levels of exposure over a short period. Acute toxicity is often caused by a chemical spill in which the exposure is sudden and often involves a large amount of the chemical. The victim may feel the effects immediately and show symptoms of dizziness, fainting, headache, nausea, and vomiting. A chronic exposure occurs with repeated lower levels of exposure over a longer period of time. The other answers do not relate to the situation described.
    CAT: Occupational Safety

76. _____ is considered regulated waste and requires special disposal.
    a. Human tissue is considered pathologic waste and requires special handling and disposal. It is categorized as infectious waste, also called regulated waste or biohazardous waste. This category includes soft tissue, extracted teeth, blood, and blood–soaked materials as well as sharps.
    CAT: Maintaining Aseptic Conditions

77. Repeated exposure to chemicals at low levels for extended periods of time can result in liver disease or brain disorders that are examples of:
    a. Chronic chemical toxicity results from many repeated exposures of lower levels over a long period of time such as months or even years. The victim may experience many effects of chronic toxicity, such as liver disease, brain disorders, cancer, or infertility. Acute chemical toxicity results from high levels of exposure over a short period.
    CAT: Occupational Safety

78. How often should a dental assistant or office safety supervisor check the contents of the emergency kit to determine that the contents are in place and within the expiration date?
    a. Because a variety of drugs may be kept in the emergency kit, many of which will

have expiration dates, the emergency kit should be checked weekly.
CAT: Occupational Safety

79. The floor in the entry to the dental office was wet. A patient slipped on the floor during entry to the office. There was no signage to include a potential slippery floor. In this case, the office owner:
    a. The office owner, whether the dentist or another building owner, must post or place signs when potential dangerous situations exist, such as the wet floor. In this case, the building owner is responsible for the placement of the sign and for the training of persons who are responsible for placing such signage.
    CAT: Patient and Dental Healthcare Worker Education

80. Wastes are classified as hazardous if they are:
    a. If a waste product is ignitable or flammable, it is considered to be hazardous, according to the EPA. The other distracters do not relate to this classification.
    CAT: Occupational Safety

81. All waste containers that hold potentially infectious materials must:
    b. Infectious waste (regulated waste) must be labeled with the universal biohazard symbol, identified in compliance with local regulations, or both. After contaminated waste leaves the office, it is then regulated by the EPA and by state and local laws.
    CAT: Occupational Safety

82. Scrap dental amalgam should be collected and stored in:
    a. Scrap dental amalgam is stored in a designated dry, airtight container. It is considered hazardous waste and poses a risk to humans and to the environment if stored otherwise.
    CAT: Occupational Safety

83. Which government agency enforces the disposal of regulated waste?
    b. The EPA is responsible for regulated waste after it leaves the dental office. The other agencies do not control the disposal of regulated waste.
    CAT: Occupational Safety

84. Which of the following does the OSHA Hazard Communications Standard require employers to do?
    d. Employers are required by the OSHA Hazard Communications Standard to tell employees about the identity and hazards of chemicals in the workplace. This agency does not make requirements dealing with employee tax records or drug or urinalysis tests.
    CAT: Occupational Safety

85. Which of the following is the dental staff required to have available and know the location of in the event of a heart attack or closed or blocked airway?
    b. Each dental health care worker must know the location of the oxygen tank in case of emergencies. Periodic updates in emergency procedures should be offered to the staff.
    CAT: Occupational Safety

86. Which of the following is *not* a requirement of hazard communication training?
    d. The waiver of hepatitis C vaccinations is not an appropriate response to hazard communication training for the dental staff. All of the other tasks are required for the employer to make available for the staff.
    CAT: Patient and Dental Healthcare Worker Education

87. A dental health care worker transfers a small amount of glass ionomer cement into a smaller container for use on a patient at chairside. A new label must be placed on that container if:
    b. If the dental cement is not used up in its entirety by the end of the work shift, an appropriate label must be attached to the bottle to meet with the requirements of the Hazard Communication Standard issued by OSHA.
    CAT: Occupational Safety

88. Hazard communication training must be provided:
    a. The Hazard Communication Standard issued by OSHA requires dentists to provide hazard communication training

to each employee at the beginning of employment and annually thereafter.
CAT: Occupational Safety

89. Which of the following is an unsafe practice when recapping the needle?
    d. The dental assistant must never use a two-handed scoop method; it is potentially dangerous because the assistant could slip and cause a needle puncture.
    CAT: Occupational Safety

90. Which of the following is *not* considered a "sharp"?
    b. The matrix retainer is not a sharp device. It is used to hold the matrix band, which is considered a sharp.
    CAT: Occupational Safety

91. Flushing the water lines of the dental unit relates to:
    c. Flushing the water lines temporarily reduces the microbial count in the water and helps to clean the handpiece waterlines of materials. Materials are flushed away, not just trapped. Temperature of the water is not an issue addressed by flushing, and flushing does not remove biofilm from the lines; biofilm can form while the water is passing through the lines.
    CAT: Asepsis Procedures

92. The ADA, OSAP, and CDC recommend that dental assistants flush the dental unit waterlines:
    b. All of the above-mentioned organizations concur that flushing of the dental unit waterlines for 30 seconds each morning and between patients will promote safe practice. This can be followed up by flushing and cleaning at the end of the day.
    CAT: Asepsis Procedures

93. Shortly after donning the required PPE, a dental health care worker notices the following symptoms: watering eyes, nasal congestion, sneezing, coughing, wheezing, shortness of breath, and even dizziness. This person may be experiencing which type of reaction?
    a. Because this condition occurred immediately upon donning the PPEs, the reaction can be identified as an immediate

hypersensitivity. A reaction like this generally occurs within 20 minutes.
CAT: Occupational Safety

94. Which of the following are the recommended five parts of the Hazard Communication Standard?
    b. According to the Hazard Communication Standard of OSHA, the five basic components are a written program, inventory of hazardous chemicals, MSDS for every chemical, proper labeling of containers, and employee training.
    CAT: Occupational Safety

95. Select the statement that is *not* true.
    c. HIV is transmitted primarily from an infected person through the following routes: intimate sexual contact, exposure to blood, blood-contaminated body fluids or blood products, or perinatal contact. The remaining statements are true.
    CAT: Patient and Dental Healthcare Worker Education

96. Switching to instruments with large, round diameters and contra-angled shanks may _____ the symptoms associated with carpal tunnel syndrome.
    a. By modifying the size and design of the instruments used at chairside, it may be possible to reduce the symptoms of carpal tunnel syndrome.
    CAT: Patient and Dental Healthcare Worker Education

97. Which of the following activities should be avoided during the use of nitrous oxide during conscious sedation?
    a. During the use of nitrous oxide, you should avoid having a conversation with the patient because this will cause movement of the nasal mask and cause potential gas leaks around the mask.
    CAT: Patient and Dental Healthcare Worker Education

98. Distillation of water is a _____ process that may remove volatile chemicals, endotoxins, and some microorganisms.
    c. The use of distilled water may ensure the elimination of volatile chemicals,

endotoxins, and some microorganisms, thus potentially providing safer water for dental office use. The other processes do not remove volatile products from water.

CAT: Instrument Processing

99. Which of the following statements is true regarding the use of biohazard warning labels?
    a. The *biohazard* label is fluorescent orange or red-orange. Labels must be on bags or sharps containers that hold potentially infectious materials, whether regulated or

nonregulated. White or green bags are not compliant in meeting the OSHA Standard for biohazard labeling.

CAT: Maintaining Aseptic Conditions

100. OSHA requires the use of standard precautions for _____.
    d. OSHA requires that standard precautions be used for all patients. Therefore, blood and other body fluids from all patients are treated as potentially infectious.

CAT: Occupational Safety

General Chairside, Radiation Health and Safety, and Infection Control

General Chairside

· ·

Directions: Select the response that best answers each of the following questions.
Only one response is correct.

1. In the Universal or Standard tooth numbering system, which letter represents the maxillary left primary second molar?
   a. K
   b. J
   c. T
   d. C

2. Which classification of carious lesions form on the occlusal surfaces or the buccal and lingual grooves of posterior teeth?
   a. Class I
   b. Class II
   c. Class III
   d. Class V

3. The more fixed attachment of the muscle that is usually the end attached to the more rigid part of the skeleton is the:
   a. origin
   b. insertion
   c. contraction
   d. infraction

4. Which of the following teeth would *not* be found in the deciduous dentition?
   a. lateral incisor
   b. canine
   c. second premolar
   d. second molar

5. What does this charting symbol indicate?
   a. missing
   b. to be extracted
   c. root canal
   d. impacted

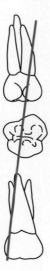

6. What does this charting symbol indicate?
   a. recurrent decay
   b. amalgam
   c. sealant
   d. missing

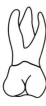

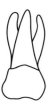

7. On a cephalometric analysis, the abbreviation Na stands for:
   a. anterior nasal spine
   b. gnathion
   c. nasion
   d. menton

8. If the charting conditions indicate that there is a furcation involvement, some type of symbol will be placed:
   a. at the apical area of the tooth
   b. on the occlusal surface of the tooth
   c. at the area between two or more root branches
   d. at the cervical region

9. What does this charting symbol indicate?
   a. gold crown
   b. stainless steel crown
   c. missing tooth
   d. post and core

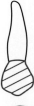

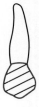

10. What does this charting symbol indicate?
   a. needs to be extracted
   b. missing tooth
   c. impacted tooth
   d. rotated tooth

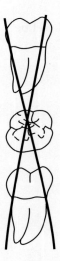

11. What does this charting symbol indicate?
   a. full crown
   b. implant
   c. root canal
   d. bonded veneer

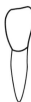

12. What does this charting symbol indicate?
   a. implant
   b. fracture
   c. diastema
   d. root canal

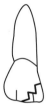

13. Which surgical procedure describes a hemisection?
   a. removal of the apical portion of the root
   b. removal of diseased tissue through scraping with a curette
   c. removal of the root and crown by cutting through each lengthwise
   d. removal of one or more roots of a multirooted tooth without removing the crown

14. How should a properly positioned dental assist be seated?
   a. on the same plane as the dentist
   b. 2 to 4 inches above the dentist
   c. 4 to 6 inches above the dentist
   d. 6 to 8 inches above the dentist

15. Using Black's classification of cavities, what class are caries along the cervical of a tooth?
   a. Class I
   b. Class II
   c. Class III
   d. Class V

16. An ML restoration on tooth #9 is classified as a _____ restoration.
   a. Class I
   b. Class II
   c. Class III
   d. Class IV
   e. Class V

17. Which instrument is used to remove subgingival calculus?
   a. curette
   b. sickle
   c. chisel
   d. hoe

18. Forceps are used in this portion of the clamp while placing the rubber dam.

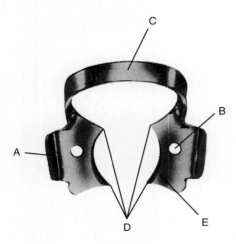

19. Which classification of motion should the dentist and the dental assistant eliminate to increase productivity and decrease stress and body fatigue?
   a. Class I
   b. Class II
   c. Class III
   d. Class IV

20. Which is an accurate statement regarding the placement of an oral evacuator tip?
   a. Place the HVE tip as far into the distal of the arch as possible.
   b. Always use the pen grasp to avoid stress on the hand.
   c. Place the angle of the HVE tip in a downward position to pick up maximum fluids.
   d. The assistant should place the HVE tip first, and then the operator should place the handpiece.

21. If a left-handed operator is preparing tooth #14 for a crown, where does the dental assistant place the bevel of the high-velocity evacuator?
   a. parallel to the buccal surface of the tooth being prepared
   b. distal to the left maxillary tuberosity from the buccal side
   c. parallel to the lingual surface of the tooth being prepared
   d. distal to the left maxillary tuberosity from the lingual side

22. Which of the following statements is *not* a concept of four-handed dentistry?
   a. Place the patient in the supine position.
   b. The operator and assistant should sit as close to the patient as possible.
   c. Use preset tray setups with instruments placed in sequence of use.
   d. Use a wide-winged patient chair back.

23. Which type of handpiece can operate both forward and backward and can be used with a variety of attachments?
 a. high speed
 b. low speed
 c. air abrasion
 d. laser

24. When a Tofflemire matrix band retainer is used, which of the knobs or devices would be used to adjust the size or loop of the matrix band to fit around the tooth and loosen the band for removal?

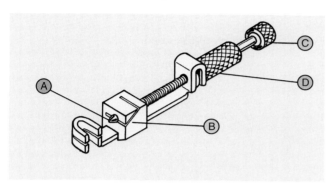

25. What is the purpose of a barbed broach?
 a. obturate the canal
 b. remove necrotic tissue
 c. place medicaments
 d. provide measurements

26. Which instrument would be used to remove debris or granulation tissue from a surgical site?
 a. rongeur forceps
 b. surgical curette
 c. bone file
 d. periosteal elevator

27. Which of the following statements is *true* regarding the use of a universal matrix band and retainer?
 a. The matrix retainer and wedge are both placed on the buccal surface.
 b. The matrix retainer is placed on the buccal surface, and the wedge is placed from the lingual at the proximal surface involved.
 c. The matrix retainer is placed on the lingual surface, and the wedge is placed from the buccal at the proximal surface involved.
 d. It is not necessary to use a wedge with a Tofflemire matrix band and retainer.

28. A dental team is restoring an MOD preparation on tooth #4 with amalgam. Which item is *not* required to place this type of restoration?
 a. wedges
 b. cleoid–discoid carver
 c. enamel hatchet
 d. Mylar matrix

29. An orthodontic positioner is designed to:
   a. move the teeth
   b. retain the teeth in their desired position
   c. reposition the teeth during orthodontic treatment
   d. support the arch wire

30. Which of these instruments would *not* be a choice when placing a gingival retraction cord?
   a. explorer
   b. cord packing instrument
   c. blunt end of a plastic instrument

31. From the photograph, what is the procedure for which this tray would be used?
   a. preparation for a cast restoration
   b. cementation of a cast restoration
   c. placement of brackets
   d. placement of separators

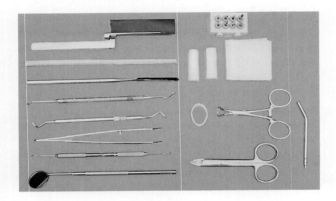

32. The instruments shown from left to right are:
   a. three-pronged pliers, posterior band remover, ligature pin, and ligature cutter
   b. Howe pliers, wire bending pliers, and ligature tying pliers
   c. bird beak pliers, contouring pliers, and Weingart utility pliers
   d. bird beak pliers, Howe pliers, and wire-bending pliers

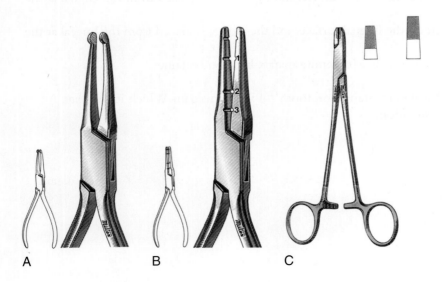

A   B   C

33. Which of the following is *not* a postoperative instruction to control bleeding after a surgical procedure?
   a. Bite on two folded gauze for at least 30 minutes after the procedure is completed.
   b. If bleeding continues and does not stop, call the dental office.
   c. Restrict strenuous work or physical activity for the remainder of the day.
   d. Rinse vigorously after 6 hours.

34. What is the endodontic test in which the dentist applies pressure to the mucosa above the apex of the root and notes any sensitivity or swelling?
   a. percussion
   b. palpation
   c. cold
   d. electric pulp vitality

35. The process by which the living jawbone naturally grows around an implanted dental supports is known as:
   a. subperiosteal implant
   b. transosteal implantation
   c. osseointegration
   d. ostectomy

36. The treatment used as an attempt to save the pulp and encourage the formation of dentin at the site of the injury is a(n):
   a. pulp capping
   b. pulpectomy
   c. apicoectomy
   d. pulpotomy

37. The removal of the coronal portion of an exposed vital pulp is a(n):
   a. pulpectomy
   b. pulpotomy
   c. apicoectomy
   d. root resection

38. The instrument used to adapt and condense gutta-percha points into the canal during endodontic treatment is:
   a. Gates Glidden bur
   b. spreader or plugger
   c. endodontic spoon excavator
   d. broach

39. The surgical removal of diseased gingival tissues is called:
   a. gingivoplasty
   b. gingivectomy
   c. osteoplasty
   d. ostectomy

40. A(n) _____ is a dentist with a license in the specialty of dentistry who provides restoration and replacement of natural teeth and supporting structures.
   a. endodontist
   b. periodontist
   c. orthodontist
   d. prosthodontist

41. Periodontal pocket depth is charted at _____ points on each tooth during a baseline charting procedure.
a. two
b. four
c. six
d. eight

42. A periodontal pocket marker is similar in design to a _____.
a. thumb forceps
b. cotton pliers
c. Gracey scaler
d. periodontal probe

43. A(n) _____ is an additive bone surgery that includes the reshaping and contouring of the bone.
a. ostectomy
b. osteoplasty
c. gingivoplasty
d. apicoectomy

44. From the instruments shown below, select the periosteal elevator.

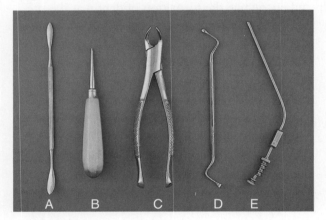

45. Using Black's classification of cavities, a pit and fissure lesion on the occlusal surface of molars and premolars is considered a Class _____ cavity.
a. I
b. II
c. III
d. V

46. Which of the following instruments would be used to transport a temporary restorative material to a cavity preparation?
a. Ward's C carver
b. #7 cleoid–discoid carver
c. explorer
d. Woodson

47. Which orthodontic pliers are used in fitting bands for fixed or removable appliances?
    a. bird beak pliers
    b. contouring pliers
    c. posterior band remover pliers
    d. Howe (110) pliers

48. Which of the following rotary instruments would cut fastest and most efficiently?
    a. tungsten carbide bur
    b. stainless steel bur
    c. diamond stone
    d. green stone

49. In selecting a shade for a composite restoration, under which of the following conditions should the shade be selected?
    a. Select before tooth preparation and dry the tooth thoroughly.
    b. Select with operating light in place before tooth preparation.
    c. Keep the tooth moist and free from bright colors.
    d. Select after tooth preparation with the tooth dried.

50. When cleaning a dental handpiece, it is important to:
    a. follow the handpiece manufacturer's directions thoroughly
    b. follow the sterilizer manufacturer's directions thoroughly
    c. always lubricate the handpiece before sterilization
    d. always lubricate the handpiece after sterilization

51. A(n) _____ procedure is performed to remove defects and to restore normal contours in the bone.
    a. gingivectomy
    b. gingivoplasty
    c. osseous surgery
    d. frenectomy

52. Which of the following is *not* a measurement used in constructing a complete denture?
    a. protrusion
    b. lateral excursion
    c. centric relation
    d. reversion

53. All of the following are categories of restorations *except:*
    a. class I
    b. class X
    c. class IV
    d. class V

54. _____ sealants _____ require mixing as they cure when they are exposed to UV light.
    a. Chemically cured, do
    b. Light cured, do
    c. Chemically cured, do not
    d. Light cured, do not

55. When adjusting a crown after cementation, the dentist most likely would use a(n) _____.
    a. diamond bur
    b. FG bur
    c. stone
    d. RA bur

56. The procedure performed to remove subgingival calculus and to remove necrotic tissue from the periodontal pocket is referred to as _____:
    a. root planing
    b. prophylaxis
    c. coronal polishing
    d. gingival curettage

57. Why would a dentist use an intraoral camera?
    a. to take a patient's picture for the dental chart
    b. to demonstrate periodontal pocket depths
    c. to gain better access to a difficult view
    d. to demonstrate proper oral hygiene

58. To minimize leakage, what would the operator do to the rubber dam around each isolated tooth?
    a. invert
    b. ligate
    c. seal
    d. punch

59. What are the attachments used for support or retention of a three-unit bridge called?
    a. pontics
    b. abutments
    c. anchors
    d. spacers

60. Which portion of the bridge replaces the missing tooth?
    a. pontic
    b. spacer
    c. anchor
    d. abutment

61. Which instrument would be passed to the operator to smooth the interproximal box on a prepared MO amalgam?
    a. a gingival margin trimmer
    b. an interproximal carver
    c. an enamel hatchet
    d. a spoon excavator

62. Which of the following would be considered a contraindication for a patient receiving a fixed bridge?
    a. controlled diabetes
    b. older than 60 years of age
    c. poor personal hygiene
    d. poor oral hygiene

63. The surgical removal of the apex of an endodontically treated tooth is what procedure?
    a. hemisection
    b. apicoectomy
    c. extraction
    d. pulpotomy

64. What is the common name for the #110 pliers?
    a. contouring pliers
    b. Howe pliers
    c. Weingart pliers
    d. band pusher

65. Before surgery, a patient is explained the procedure and then signs an authorization for treatment. What is this process called?
    a. implied consent
    b. informed consent
    c. release of information
    d. authorization for treatment

66. A patient who is said to be "tongue tied" would have what type of procedure?
    a. osteotomy
    b. frenectomy
    c. alveoplasty
    d. ostectomy

67. The water-to-powder ratio generally used for an adult maxillary impression is _____ measures of water and _____ scoops of powder.
    a. 3, 3
    b. 3, 2
    c. 3, 4
    d. 2, 2

68. If using a self-cure composite resin system, what will occur if the containers are cross-contaminated?
    a. It will cause the material to harden.
    b. It will prevent the material from hardening.
    c. The translucency will be diminished.
    d. Polymerization will be delayed.

69. Which statement is incorrect regarding tooth conditioner?
    a. The conditioning agent forms a mechanical bond with the enamel.
    b. The conditioning agent is flooded onto the surface and rubbed vigorously.
    c. The conditioning agent is generally applied with special applicators provided by the manufacturer.
    d. The conditioning agent is rinsed from the tooth after a recommended time to stop the etching process.

70. Which of the following materials would *not* be used to take a final impression for the creation of a prosthetic device?
    a. silicone
    b. polysiloxane
    c. alginate hydrocolloid
    d. agar hydrocolloid

71. A porcelain fused to a metal crown would be designed so the porcelain would always be on which surface?
a. lingual
b. facial
c. mesial
d. distal

72. A glass ionomer material may be used for all of the following *except* a(n):
a. restorative material
b. liner
c. luting agent
d. obtundant

73. If the room temperature and humidity are very low while mixing a final impression material, the setting time may be:
a. decreased
b. increased

74. A porcelain fused to a metal crown is being seated. The assistant will mix the cement to a _____ or _____ consistency.
a. base, secondary
b. luting, secondary
c. base, primary
d. luting, primary

75. A posterior tooth with a deep preparation may require a base that is designed to prepare pulpal defense by functioning as a(n):
a. final restoration
b. protective base
c. insulating base
d. sedative base

76. IRM (intermediate restorative material) is used primarily for:
a. final restorative for primary molars
b. provisional restoration
c. cementing crowns, bridges, and onlays
d. seating an implant

77. A patient has a fractured amalgam on 29DO. Time in the doctor's schedule does not permit placement of a permanent restoration. Which of the following statements is *correct* as to the type of dental cement and the consistency that would be used in this clinical situation?
a. temporary cement to a secondary consistency
b. final cement to a secondary consistency
c. temporary cement to a primary consistency
d. final cement to a primary consistency

78. A reproduction of an individual tooth on which a wax pattern may be constructed for a cast crown is a(n):
a. die
b. model
c. cast
d. impression

79. Which food can be compared to a reversible hydrocolloid?
   a. potato chips
   b. salad dressing
   c. ice cream
   d. ketchup

80. An alginate impression has been taken to prepare a set of diagnostic models. Which of the following statements is *false* as it relates to handling the impression? Alginate impressions _____.
   a. should be stored for as short a period as possible
   b. expand when stored in water
   c. shrink when stored in air with low humidity
   d. can be stored in 100% relative humidity without serious dimensional changes for up to 24 hours

81. A broken removable denture prosthesis can be repaired:
   a. at home by the patient with an OTC kit
   b. at home by the patient with superglue
   c. in the office with cold-cured acrylic
   d. in the office with light-cured composite

82. A removable denture prosthesis can be cleaned in the dental office by all of the methods listed below *except:*
   a. immersion in an ultrasonic cleaner with a special denture cleaning solution
   b. brushing with a denture brush
   c. removing calculus with hand instruments
   d. with routine prophylaxis instruments and brushes in the patient's mouth

83. A patient is seen early in the morning. The record indicates she has diabetes. She mentions she had not yet had breakfast but took all of her medications before the appointment. As the appointment progresses, it is noted that she is perspiring, seems not able to focus on conversation, and is increasingly anxious. These symptoms are an indication of:
   a. angina attack
   b. hyperventilation
   c. hyperglycemia
   d. hypoglycemia

84. Which of the following statements is *not* true as it relates to a patient's respiration?
   a. If a patient knows the breaths are being monitored, he or she will usually change the breathing pattern.
   b. For children and teenagers, the respiration rate is higher than that of an adult.
   c. A person's respiration normally is not noticeable unless he or she is having trouble taking a breath.
   d. Respirations are normally higher in counts per minute than the pulse rate.

85. What is the respiration pattern for a patient in a state of tachypnea?
   a. a slow respiration rate
   b. excessively short, rapid breaths
   c. excessively long, rapid breaths
   d. a gurgling sound

86. What is the respiration pattern for a patient who is hyperventilating?
    a. a slow respiration rate
    b. excessively short, rapid breaths
    c. excessively long, rapid breaths
    d. a gurgling sound

87. In an emergency the staff member should feel for the pulse of a conscious patient at which artery?
    a. brachial
    b. femoral
    c. radial
    d. carotid

88. If a patient displays symptoms of hyperglycemia and is conscious, what is the first thing you should ask the patient?
    a. "What time did you awaken this morning?"
    b. "When did you last eat?"
    c. "How many fingers do you see?" while holding up your fingers.
    d. "Did you bring a snack?"

89. Which of the following are the recommended guidelines for cardiopulmonary resuscitation?
    a. access, breathing, and circulation,
    b. access, breathing, circulation, and defibrillation
    c. airway, breathing, and compressions
    d. compressions, airway, and breathing

90. Which of the following conditions is *not* a potential medical contraindication to nitrous oxide?
    a. nasal obstruction
    b. emphysema and multiple sclerosis
    c. emotional instability
    d. age

91. What substance is added to a local anesthetic agent to slow down the intake of the agent and increase the duration of action?
    a. sodium chloride
    b. a vasoconstrictor
    c. an amide
    d. an ester

92. The type of anesthesia achieved by injecting the anesthetic solution directly into the tissue at the site of the dental procedure is known as _____.
    a. inferior alveolar nerve block anesthesia
    b. field block anesthesia
    c. infiltration anesthesia
    d. anterior palatine nerve block

93. General anesthesia is most safely administered in a:
    a. general dentist's office
    b. hospital or oral surgeon's office
    c. pedodontist's office
    d. periodontist's office

94. Which of the following refers to an allergic response that could threaten the patient's life?
   a. grand mal
   b. myocardial infarction
   c. anaphylaxis
   d. hypersensitivity

95. How should the staff respond if a patient is having a grand mal seizure?
   a. Stand back and let the seizure run its course.
   b. Place the patient in an upright and seated position.
   c. Clear away any hazards and call EMS.
   d. Try to open the patient's airway.

96. In which situation is nitroglycerin placed under the tongue of a patient?
   a. heart failure
   b. angina
   c. cerebrovascular accident
   d. severe allergic reaction

97. MyPlate is an outline of what to eat each day. The smallest segment of the plate concept represents which food source?
   a. grains
   b. vegetables
   c. meats
   d. oils

98. How are foods that contain sugars or other carbohydrates that can be metabolized by bacteria in plaque categorized?
   a. cariostatic
   b. cariogenic
   c. composed of empty calories
   d. complex carbohydrate

99. Organic substances that occur in plant and animal tissues are _____, and essential elements that are needed in small amounts to maintain health and function are _____.
   a. minerals, vitamins
   b. fat-soluble vitamins, water-soluble vitamins
   c. vitamins, minerals
   d. cholesterol, minerals

100. Dry mouth is also known as _____.
   a. periodontal disease
   b. blastoma
   c. xerostomia
   d. glossitis

101. _____is more prominent in older adults who have experienced gingival recession.
   a. Interproximal dental decay
   b. Cervical caries
   c. Incisal caries
   d. Generalized dental decay

102. Which factor would *not* contribute to xerostomia in a patient?
   a. disease processes
   b. dietary intake
   c. medications
   d. age

103. Which of the following would *not* be suggested as an intervention for the prevention of dental caries?
   a. fluoride
   b. antibacterial therapy
   c. decreased ingestion of carbohydrates
   d. chewing mints

104. A caries risk assessment test is used to determine the _____.
   a. number of mutans streptococci and lactobacilli present in the saliva
   b. amount of fermentable carbohydrate present in the saliva
   c. level of salivary immunity
   d. salinity of the saliva

105. Inflammation of the supporting tissues of the teeth that begins with _____ can progress into the connective tissue and alveolar bone that supports the teeth and become _____.
   a. gingivitis, glossitis
   b. periodontitis, gingivitis
   c. gingivitis, periodontitis
   d. gingivitis, gangrene

106. A dietary food analysis includes a diary of everything a patient consumes for:
   a. 24 hours
   b. 72 hours
   c. 1 week
   d. 1 month

107. MyPlate is an outline of what to eat each day. Which of the following statements is *true* regarding MyPlate?
   a. MyPlate includes a base formed of dairy products.
   b. The smallest portion of MyPlate is composed of fats products.
   c. Recent research supports MyPlate for a vegetarian diet.
   d. The MyPlate concept has no scientific validity.

108. The patient's record indicates that the status of the gingiva is bulbous, flattened, punched out, and cratered. This statement describes the gingival _____:
   a. color
   b. contour
   c. consistency
   d. surface texture

109. When transferring patient records from the office to another site, the administrative assistant must do all *except* which of the following?
   a. Obtain consent from the patient or legal representative.
   b. Retain the original record in the office.
   c. Transfer the entire record.
   d. Copy the radiographs and retain the originals.

110. A new filing system for clinical charts is to be installed in the office. Which of the following filing systems would be most efficient?
    a. open files with colored filing labels with alpha and numeric codes
    b. vertical files with tab-top labels
    c. vertical files with closed-end folders
    d. lateral files with closed-end folders

111. If an administrative assistant chooses to transmit a transaction about a patient electronically, under which Act does this task fall?
    a. ADA
    b. HHS
    c. HIPAA
    d. NIOSH

112. A message about a serious illness or allergy should be noted in which manner on the clinical record?
    a. on the outside of the record in a large, bright color
    b. inside the record in a discreet but obvious manner such as a small, brightly colored label
    c. in large print on the lower-right edge of the outside of the record
    d. in large print inside the record

113. The group responsible for establishing regulations that govern the practice of dentistry within a state is the:
    a. American Dental Association
    b. Dental Assisting National Board
    c. Commission on Dental Accreditation
    d. Board of Dentistry

114. The act of doing something that a reasonably prudent person would not do or not doing something that a reasonably prudent person would do is:
    a. fraud
    b. abandonment
    c. negligence
    d. defamation of character

115. A clinical dental assistant is hired in the practice. The dentist indicates that this person is to place an intracoronal provisional restoration. The person knows how to perform the task but does not yet have the EFDA credential required to perform the specific intraoral task. What should the new employee do?
    a. Do what the dentist told her to do.
    b. Perform the task now but later tell the dentist that he or she does not have the appropriate credential.
    c. Inform the dentist that he or she does not yet have the appropriate credential to perform the task.
    d. Perform the task with the self-assurance that he or she will soon have the credential.

116. The Good Samaritan Law offers incentives for health care providers to provide medical assistance to injured persons without the fear of potential litigation except under which of the following circumstances?
    a. protection for a negligent health care provider who is being compensated for services
    b. immunity for acts performed by a person who renders care in an emergency situation
    c. when the provider is solely interested in providing care in a safe manner with no intent to do bodily harm

117. The objectives of good appointment book management include all *except* which of the following?
   a. Maximize productivity.
   b. Reduce staff tension.
   c. Maintain concern for the patients' needs.
   d. Allow for maximum downtime.

118. In reference to appointment management, *prime time* refers to:
   a. the time during which the dentist performs the most expensive type of treatment
   b. the time most frequently requested by patients
   c. the first 2 hours of the daily schedule
   d. midday appointment times

119. Which time of day is considered most appropriate when treating young children?
   a. just before naptime
   b. immediately after naptime
   c. early morning
   d. late in the day

120. What type of supply is a curing light used in the treatment room?
   a. expendable
   b. nonexpendable
   c. capital
   d. variable

Radiation Health and Safety

Directions: Select the response that best answers each of the following questions. Only one response is correct.

1. What is the appearance of a bent film?
   a. Herringbone pattern on the film
   b. Black lines in the corners of the film
   c. White lines in the corners of the film
   d. Thin, black branching lines across the film

2. What is the correction for an image that is foreshortened?
   a. Increase the vertical angulation.
   b. Adjust the horizontal angulation.
   c. Decrease the vertical angulation.
   d. Ask the patient to lift up his or her chin during exposure.

3. What is the most common reason to see a completely clear film?
   a. Film was exposed to light.
   b. Film was not exposed to x-radiation.
   c. Film was exposed backwards in the mouth.
   d. Film was placed in fixer before developer solution.

4. Why is the use of a thyroid collar discouraged in panoramic radiography?
   a. It cannot be disinfected.
   b. It blocks a portion of the x-ray beam.
   c. It affects the positioning of the Frankfort plane.
   d. Together with the lead apron, the thyroid collar is too heavy for the patient.

5. Which radiographic technique provides the most accurate representation of the tooth and surrounding structures?
   a. Bite-wing
   b. Paralleling
   c. Panoramic
   d. Bisecting angle

6. The silver halide crystals are found in what component of the x-ray film?
   a. Film base
   b. Adhesive layer
   c. Film emulsion
   d. Protective layer

7. All of the following can be found in the cathode except one. Which is the EXCEPTION?
   a. Tungsten target
   b. Molybdenum cup
   c. Tungsten filament
   d. Negatively charged electrode

8. What is the penetrating x-ray beam that exits the tubehead?
   a. Primary beam
   b. Scatter radiation
   c. Secondary radiation
   d. Characteristic radiation

9. X-rays are produced at the:
   a. positive anode.
   b. negative anode.
   c. positive cathode.
   d. negative cathode.

10. What process is occurring in this image?
    a. External resorption
    b. Physiologic resorption
    c. Internal resorption
    d. Ectopic eruption

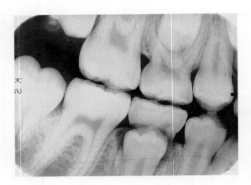

11. What is the radiopaque restoration in this image?
    a. A composite restoration with an overhang on the mesial surface
    b. An amalgam restoration with an overhang on the mesial surface
    c. A composite restoration with an overhang on the distal surface
    d. An amalgam restoration with an overhang on the distal surface

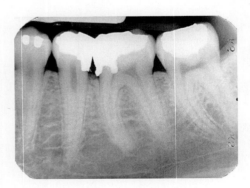

12. What landmark is indicated by the arrows?
   a. Coronoid process
   b. Condyle
   c. Internal oblique ridge
   d. Zygomatic process of the maxilla

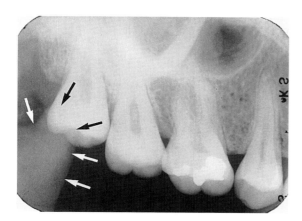

13. What type of radiograph is preferred to evaluate for an incisal crown fracture?
   a. Occlusal
   b. Bite-wing
   c. Periapical
   d. Panoramic

14. Which of the following steps should be followed when exposing a panoramic radiograph?
   a. Place a lead apron with a thyroid collar on the patient and secure it.
   b. Instruct the patient to place his or her posterior teeth in the deep groove on the bite block and bite firmly.
   c. Radiodense objects may remain in place from the head and neck area for the duration of the exposure.
   d. Instruct the patient to close the lips on the bite block and to swallow once and then place the tongue against the roof of the mouth to maintain that position during exposure.

15. To expose bite-wing radiographs, which size or sizes of receptors are used?
   a. 0, 1, 2
   b. 0, 2, 3
   c. 0, 1, 2, 3, 4
   d. 4 only

16. Which is NOT an accurate definition used in dental radiography?
   a. Parallel: always separated by the same distance
   b. Intersecting: to cut through
   c. Right angle: formed by two parallel lines
   d. Central ray: central portion of the beam

17. Optimum time and temperature for manual processing is _____.
   a. 62 degrees at 5½ minutes
   b. 64 degrees at 6½ minutes
   c. 66 degrees at 3½ minutes
   d. 68 degrees at 4½ minutes

18. Which component of the x-ray film packet should be recycled?
    a. Film
    b. Lead foil
    c. Black paper
    d. Outer package wrapping

19. If films are left in the fixer solution for 9 minutes, approximately how much time is spent in the developer solution?
    a. 3.0 minutes
    b. 3.5 minutes
    c. 4.0 minutes
    d. 4.5 minutes

20. What is the purpose of a step wedge radiograph?
    a. To check the film speed
    b. To examine the darkroom for light leaks
    c. To ensure the strength of the processing solutions
    d. To maintain the settings on the exposure control panel

21. When mounting a full mouth series, it is recommended to begin with which films?
    a. Bite-wings
    b. Maxillary anterior periapicals
    c. Mandibular anterior periapicals
    d. Mandibular posterior periapicals

22. Which statements are true about the lead apron?
    a. A lead apron must always be attached.
    b. A lead apron should never be folded for storage.
    c. A lead apron should be stored hanging up.
    d. Both b and c are true.

23. Which cell would be considered to have high radiation sensitivity?
    a. Liver
    b. Nerve
    c. Salivary gland
    d. Small lymphocyte

24. When a radiographer is producing a radiographic image on a patient, it is recommended that the radiographer stand in which direction from the primary beam?
    a. Straight line
    b. Any direction
    c. Perpendicular
    d. One step outside the operatory

25. What is the maximum permissible dose an occupationally exposed pregnant individual is allowed to accumulate in a year?
    a. 5.0 rem
    b. 1.0 rem
    c. 0.1 rem
    d. 0.01 rem

26. If a radiographer cannot stand 6 feet away from the primary beam, which of the following should he or she do?
    a. Wear a lead apron when exposing radiographs.
    b. Stand behind a lead-lined wall.
    c. Do not take an image.
    d. No additional precautions need to be made.

27. When the dental assistant becomes the patient, where is the radiation-monitoring badge placed?
    a. Cover it with the lead apron.
    b. Wear it at waist level as always.
    c. Place it in a drawer inside the radiology cubicle.
    d. Leave it in a radiation-safe area outside of the radiology cubicle.

28. Which of the following relates to patient safety?
    a. Leakage from the tubehead
    b. Distance from the source
    c. Concrete walls
    d. Paralleling technique

29. Which of the following is a safety concern for the operator?
    a. Thickness of the filter
    b. Use of a thyroid collar
    c. Somatic effects
    d. Thermionic emission

30. Which radiographic exposure is the best choice for the intraoral examination of large areas of the upper or lower jaw?
    a. Occlusal
    b. Periapical
    c. Bite-wing
    d. Panoramic

31. When would tomography be used in dentistry?
    a. Silography
    b. Digital radiography
    c. Scanning of the temporomandibular joint (TMJ)

32. Which statement is NOT true about a bite-wing radiograph?
    a. The receptor is placed in the mouth parallel to the crowns of both the upper and lower teeth.
    b. The receptor is stabilized when the patient bites on the bite-wing tab or bite-wing receptor holder.
    c. The central ray of the x-ray beam is directed through the contacts of the teeth using a vertical angulation of +40 degrees.
    d. The bite-wing radiograph is a method used to examine the interproximal surfaces of the teeth.

33. What will occur when voltage is increased?
    a. Electrons move from the anode to the cathode with more speed.
    b. Photons move from the anode to the cathode with more speed.
    c. Electrons move from the cathode to the anode with more speed.
    d. Photons move from the cathode to the anode with more speed.

34. With faster F-speed film, a single intraoral film results in a surface skin exposure of _____ milliroentgens.
    a. 1.25
    b. 12.5
    c. 100
    d. 250

35. Quality control tests that should be applied to dental office radiology standards should include which procedure?
    a. Regular maintenance
    b. Logging the number of images taken
    c. Evaluating the operator's technique
    d. Exposing images on a staff member to check quality

36. In which exposure will the genial tubercle be seen?
    a. Maxillary central
    b. Mandibular central
    c. Maxillary molar
    d. Mandibular molar

37. What will occur if a lead apron is folded instead of hung?
    a. It will shred and mold.
    b. It will crack and become ineffective.
    c. It will gradually fall apart and become powdery.
    d. It will crack and remain effective.

38. Which type of radiation byproduct is NOT associated with patient interaction?
    a. Primary
    b. Secondary
    c. Tertiary
    d. Scatter

39. Which type of lead apron should be used when exposing a panoramic radiograph?
    a. Single-sided apron with a thyroid collar
    b. Single-sided apron without a thyroid collar
    c. Double-sided apron with a thyroid collar
    d. Double-sided apron without a thyroid collar

40. Which type of radiation is the penetrating x-ray beam that is produced at the target of the anode?
    a. Scatter
    b. Particulate
    c. Primary
    d. Leakage

41. Which statement would NOT be a function of the Consumer-Patient Radiation Health and Safety Act?
    a. Mandating the number of radiographic exposures for specific treatment
    b. Establishing guidelines for the proper maintenance of x-ray equipment
    c. Requiring persons who take dental radiographs to be properly trained and certified
    d. Outlining requirements for the safe use of dental x-ray equipment

42. Which term best describes the concept of radiation protection as it pertains to technique, amount, and quality?
   a. ALARA
   b. Bremsstrahlung
   c. Joule
   d. Rogerian

43. The lack of which of the following actions could constitute patient negligence?
   a. Informed consent
   b. Common law
   c. Statutory law
   d. Standards of care

44. What is the best way to limit a patient's radiation exposure?
   a. Prescribe only what is necessary.
   b. Use the fastest speed film available.
   c. Complete films with no errors.
   d. Wear a lead apron.

45. Under which situation is it NOT necessary for the patient to wear a thyroid collar?
   a. If the thyroid collar gets in the way of an accurate intraoral radiograph
   b. If the patient is having trouble tolerating the weight around the neck
   c. If the patient is currently on thyroid medication
   d. During extraoral exposures

46. What is the maximum permissible dose radiation for occupationally exposed workers?
   a. 2 rem/yr
   b. 5 rem/yr
   c. 10 rem/yr
   d. 25 rem/yr

47. What is a practical alternative for operator safety in the absence of a lead wall?
   a. The operator stands at a 45-degree angle to the tubehead.
   b. The operator stands at a 90-degree angle to the tubehead.
   c. The operator stands behind the tubehead.
   d. The operator wears a lead apron for all exposures.

48. Which agency regulates the manufacture and installation of dental x-ray equipment?
   a. The local government
   b. The municipality
   c. The state government
   d. The federal government

49. Which factor is used to measure the penetrating power of radiation?
   a. Velocity
   b. Wavelength
   c. Amplitude
   d. Frequency

50. Which body tissue listed is the least sensitive to radiation exposure?
    a. Small blood vessels
    b. Bone marrow
    c. Thyroid gland
    d. Lymph glands

51. What is the maximum permissible dose of radiation for a pregnant patient?
    a. 0.1 rem/9 mo
    b. 0.8 rem/9 mo
    c. 1.0 rem/9 mo
    d. 5.0 rem/9 mo

52. Which situation could be used as an exception to placing the operator in the path of the primary beam?
    a. The patient is unable to tolerate a receptor holder.
    b. The tubehead is drifting.
    c. The child patient has had trauma and is uncooperative.
    d. There is no exception to this rule.

53. When x-ray exposure time is increased, there is _____ density of the radiograph.
    a. increased
    b. decreased

54. One reason patients object to having dental radiographs taken is_____.
    a. lack of information as to the value
    b. that X-radiation is dangerous
    c. because the patient cannot take radiographs home
    d. that insurance will not pay for them

55. Misleading information as to the value of dental radiographs is from which of the following source?
    a. Peer-reviewed journals
    b. *Journal of the American Dental Association*
    c. Popular magazines
    d. ADA Council on Dental Education

56. When asked by a patient about a dark area appearing at the root of a tooth, the response of the dental assistant should be which of the following?
    a. Tell the patient it is probably an abscess.
    b. Tell the patient it is probably an artifact on the image.
    c. Tell the patient the dentist will explain all findings.
    d. Tell the patient it is nothing to worry about.

57. Proper chair adjustment for dental radiographs is which of the following?
    a. Upright with headrest supporting the occipital lobe at -10 degrees
    b. Upright
    c. Slightly reclined at 10 degrees.
    d. Slightly reclined at 15 degrees.

58. Improperly stored film will appear _____.
  a. fogged
  b. light
  c. striped
  d. with light bars at the edges

59. Correct solution maintenance for manual film processing includes
_____.
  a. changing both developer and fixer at the same time
  b. diluting fixer to keep the level at optimal levels
  c. never adding new solutions to the developer or fixer until they are ready to be completely changed
  d. replacing the developer solution if the image appears yellow

60. _____results in deposits appearing on the walls of the processing tank.
  a. Precipitation from hard water
  b. A buildup of silver salts
  c. Reaction of the mineral salts in the water and carbonate in the processing solutions
  d. Contaminated solutions

61. Dental x-ray film has the following properties EXCEPT: _____.
  a. a specific infection protocol for exposing
  b. a specific infection protocol for the developing process
  c. a specific storage requirement
  d. a long shelf life if stored properly

62. Optimal humidity in an area storing dental film is: _____.
  a. 25% –29%
  b. 30% –50%
  c. 55% –63%
  d. 63% –68%

63. A breakdown of chemicals in the processing solution that results from air exposure is the definition of which of the following terms?
  a. Contamination
  b. Reduction
  c. Exhaustion
  d. Oxidation

64. Of the following, which is added to the processing solution to compensate for oxidation?
  a. Acidifier
  b. Hardener
  c. Preservative
  d. Restrainer

65. Rinsing dental film in the manual development process accomplishes which of the following?
  a. Removes the silver halide crystals from the emulsion
  b. Slows down the fixation process
  c. Removes the developer and fixer solutions from the films
  d. Removes developer solution from the film and stops the development process

66. A film that is exposed too closely to a safelight filter will appear _____.
    a. fogged
    b. blurred
    c. very dark
    d. very light

67. The film required for film duplication is called by which of the following terms?
    a. Panoramic film
    b. Augmentation film
    c. Duplication film
    d. Double film

68. Film duplication can be accomplished with the use of _____.
    a. an automatic processor only
    b. a manual processor only
    c. either an automatic processor or a manual processor

69. It is best to retain dental records for at least _____ years.
    a. 3
    b. 5
    c. 7
    d. 10

70. Used developer solution is considered _____.
    a. hazardous waste
    b. flammable
    c. combustible
    d. nonhazardous waste

71. Fixer solution and rinse water can be discharged into sanitary drain systems when

    _____.
    a. the solutions have evaporated by half
    b. the temperature is equal to that of the room
    c. all of the silver has been removed
    d. they are mixed with equal parts of distilled water

72. Undeveloped dental film must be disposed of in which of the following ways?
    a. Placed in normal office waste receptacle
    b. Placed in a specified area, kept for 6 years, then discarded in regular trash
    c. Shredded and placed in a biohazard bag
    d. Collected by an approved waste removal service

73. Recycled radiographic material includes all of the following EXCEPT _____.
    a. Silver removed from fixer solution
    b. Lead foil
    c. Black paper wrapper

74. All employers must comply with OSHA Standards for Workplace Safety under which of the following conditions?
    a. An employer is under no obligation to comply with the OSHA Standard for Workplace Safety.
    b. If the office has at least 6 staff members, it must comply.
    c. If the staff working are licensed dental professionals, the office must comply.
    d. Regardless of the number of employees, all employers must comply with OSHA Standard for Workplace Safety.

75. OSHA guidelines must be adhered to by which of the following?
    a. The dentist only
    b. Only those employees handling hazardous materials
    c. All staff with the exception of the font desk
    d. All employees

76. All Safety Data Sheets must be _____.
    a. maintained on site and supplied by the manufacturer
    b. in place once the product has been opened and used once
    c. kept in a notebook and can be kept offsite for updating
    d. accessed online

77. Which type of material can transmit germs or certain diseases?
    a. Communicable
    b. Infectious
    c. Hazardous
    d. Reactive

78. Processing solutions are available in all EXCEPT which of the following forms?
    a. Powder
    b. Vacuum-packed
    c. Ready-to-use liquid
    d. Liquid concentrate

79. EPA-registered chemical germicides labeled as *hospital disinfectants* are classified as _____.
    a. high-level disinfectants
    b. intermediate-level disinfectants
    c. low-level disinfectants

80. Dental darkrooms should be disinfected with a/an _____.
    a. high-level disinfectant
    b. intermediate-level disinfectant
    c. low-level disinfectant

81. Adjusting the chair and headrest, placing the lead apron, and removing metal objects from the head and neck area on a patient should be completed by the dental professional _____.
    a. before washing hands, prior to gloving
    b. after gloving
    c. after gloving and over gloving with vinyl gloves
    d. wearing utility gloves

82. Films removed from the film packet that have not been in a barrier envelope are processed in a daylight loader with _____.
    a. gloved hands
    b. ungloved hands
    c. hands with powder-free gloves
    d. hands with utility gloves

83. Which describes how a dental radiography film should be dispensed?
    a. Counted out and placed on the bracket tray
    b. Centrally dispensed in a cup
    c. Centrally dispensed in an envelope
    d. Placed in the chart and carried into the radiography room

84. Which best describes the function of a plastic barrier cover for a digital radiography sensor?
    a. The barrier allows the sensor to be reused easily without disinfection.
    b. The barrier cover protects the sensor from chemical erosion.
    c. The barrier keeps the positioning device in line with the top of the sensor.
    d. The barrier protects the sensor from saliva contamination.

85. After each use, before processing, each receptor must be _____.
    a. disinfected
    b. dried with a paper towel
    c. decontaminated
    d. wiped with alcohol between use

86. Who determines the hazards of a chemical?
    a. The hazardous waste removal facility
    b. OSHA
    c. The employer
    d. OSAP

87. Washing with a nonantimicrobial soap and water describes which term?
    a. Standard handwashing
    b. Antiseptic handwashing
    c. Routine handwashing
    d. Antiseptic hand rub

88. Which of the following statements regarding personal protective equipment (PPE) with radiography procedures is INCORRECT?
    a. PPE must be discarded after every patient contact.
    b. PPE must be removed before leaving the dental office.
    c. PPE must be worn by all dental professionals.
    d. PPE must be worn to prevent contact with infectious materials

89. An instrument that does not contact mucous membranes is considered a _____ instrument.
    a. critical
    b. semicritical
    c. noncritical
    d. semicritical and noncritical

90. Receptors collected from a series of radiographs must be placed in a receptacle bearing the patient's name. The operator should be _____.
    a. gloved
    b. ungloved
    c. gloved with powder-free gloves

91. Spatter of blood or saliva is not routinely associated with the exposure or processing of dental images.
    a. True; therefore, minimal infection control procedures apply.
    b. True; however, transmission of infectious diseases is still possible.
    c. False; spatter is routinely experienced while processing dental images.
    d. True; therefore, operators do not need to be concerned about PPE.

92. Which infection control practice in the dental health care setting applies to radiography procedures?
    a. Vaccinations required of dental professionals
    b. Dental unit and environmental surface disinfection
    c. Exposed dental film disinfection prior to developing
    d. PPE discarded at the conclusion of the appointment

93. Which procedure must be prepared prior to seating the patient?
    a. Removal of metal objects from the patient's head and neck area
    b. Image receptors
    c. Beam alignment devices
    d. A, B, and C

94. Which of the following occurs after glove removal?
    a. Transfer of beam alignment device to the countertop
    b. Disposal of all contaminated items
    c. Removal of the lead apron
    d. Placement of the beam alignment device in area for disassembly

95. A commercially available plastic sleeve that fits over intraoral films is called a _____.
    a. plastic barrier
    b. plastic sleeve
    c. baggie
    d. tube

96. Which choice describes infection control protocol for an interrupted radiographic procedure?
    a. Removing gloves and upon return, re-gloving with the same gloves
    b. Overgloving with latex gloves and upon return, removing the outer gloves
    c. Removing gloves, washing hands, and upon return, washing hands and regloving
    d. None of the above

97. Which choice would be included in the benefits involved in the use of surface barriers?
    a. Faster room turnaround time
    b. Minimization of the use of disinfectant sprays
    c. Ease of application
    d. A, B, and C
    e. A and B

98. Which is the final step in handling film with barrier envelopes during processing?
  a. Allow the film to drop on a paper towel.
  b. Wipe each film with disinfectant.
  c. Unwrap and process films.
  d. Dispose of barrier envelopes.

99. Which of the following is the LEAST in concerns related to infection control in a radiographic procedure?
  a. Water line biofilm
  b. Direct transmission of pathogens
  c. Indirect transmission of pathogens
  d. Aerosolization

100. Which structure appears in this panoramic image?
  a. Orthodontic appliances
  b. Orthodontic bands
  c. Metal framework for two partial dentures
  d. Fused gold crowns

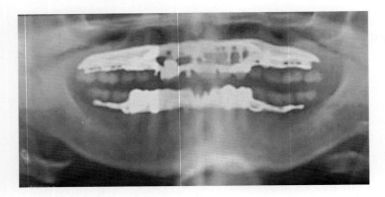

Infection Control

Directions: Select the response that best answers each of the following questions. Only one response is correct.

1. Which federal agency requires employers to inform employees of their risk regarding bloodborne pathogens?
   a. Centers for Disease Control and Prevention (CDC)
   b. Occupational Safety and Health Administration (OSHA)
   c. Food and Drug Administration (FDA)
   d. Environmental Protection Agency (EPA)

2. According to OSHA, which type of control is responsible for reducing the risk of bloodborne pathogens in the workplace by confining or isolating infectious materials?
   a. administrative
   b. work practice
   c. engineering
   d. housekeeping

3. After initial training, how often should employees receive training concerning the OSHA Bloodborne Pathogens Standard?
   a. monthly
   b. twice a year
   c. at least annually
   d. only if needed

4. According to the Hazard Communication Standard, when should established employees receive training in hazard chemicals?
   a. at least weekly
   b. upon introduction of a new hazard
   c. every month
   d. every other year

5. Which type of microorganism is the smallest?
   a. cocci
   b. viruses
   c. yeasts
   d. bacilli

6. What is the purpose of the Hazard Communication Standard?
   a. provide patients with information concerning their care
   b. inform employees of their chemical risks at work
   c. provide the public with chemical safety information
   d. help manufacturers improve their MSDS

7. Who is responsible for providing MSDS?
   a. employer
   b. dental supply company
   c. OSHA
   d. chemical's manufacturer

8. With which hazards does section III of an MSDS deal?
   a. hazardous ingredients
   b. fire or explosion hazards
   c. health hazards
   d. physical hazards

9. Which factor contributes to the growth of biofilm in dental unit water lines?
   a. using an enzymatic leaner
   b. low water temperature
   c. refillable water source
   d. standing water in the lines

10. Which type of immunity is passed from mother to child in the womb?
    a. active
    b. artificial passive
    c. natural passive
    d. acquired

11. Which government agency requires employers to protect their employees from exposure to patient blood and other body fluids?
    a. Environmental Protection Agency (EPA)
    b. Centers for Disease Control and Prevention (CDC)
    c. Food and Drug Administration (FDA)
    d. Occupational Safety and Health Administration (OSHA)

12. Which government agency regulates the effectiveness of sterilizers?
    a. Environmental Protection Agency (EPA)
    b. Centers for Disease Control and Prevention (CDC)
    c. Food and Drug Administration (FDA)
    d. Occupational Safety and Health Administration (OSHA)

13. Which government agency regulates surface disinfectants?
    a. Environmental Protection Agency (EPA)
    b. Centers for Disease Control and Prevention (CDC)
    c. Food and Drug Administration (FDA)
    d. Occupational Safety and Health Administration (OSHA)

14. Biofilm in dental unit water lines could contaminate dental personnel through which method?
    a. aerosols
    b. sharps injury
    c. direct contact
    d. cross-contamination

15. Which agency is dedicated to infection control in dentistry?
    a. Association for Advancement of Medical Instrumentation
    b. American Dental Assistants Association
    c. Organization for Safety and Asepsis Procedures
    d. Association of Professionals in Infection Control and Epidemiology

16. Extracted teeth are considered what type of waste?
    a. infectious
    b. common
    c. toxic
    d. hazardous

17. When are opportunistic infections most likely to strike?
    a. when a person is recovering from infection
    b. when a person has a chronic infection
    c. when a person has a latent infection
    d. when a person has an acute infection

18. How often should dental health care workers receive the influenza vaccine?
    a. once
    b. twice a year
    c. once a year
    d. every 10 years

19. Which method is *not* recommended for sterilizing handpieces?
    a. steam under pressure
    b. flash processing
    c. cold chemical/immersion
    d. dry heat

20. How often should one receive the tetanus vaccine?
    a. once a year
    b. every 2 years
    c. every 5 years
    d. every 10 years

21. Who is responsible for paying the cost of vaccinating at-risk employees against hepatitis B?
    a. the employee
    b. the employer
    c. insurance company
    d. the federal government

22. For which illness is there currently no available vaccine?
    a. varicella
    b. hepatitis C
    c. influenza
    d. mumps

23. What is the last piece of personal protective equipment put on before treating a patient?
    a. mask
    b. clinical gown
    c. protective eyewear
    d. gloves

24. What is the first piece of personal protective equipment taken off after treating a patient?
    a. mask
    b. clinical gown
    c. protective eyewear
    d. gloves

25. Which type of gloves should one wear when assisting during the placement of an amalgam?
    a. sterile surgical
    b. utility
    c. examination
    d. nonmedical

26. Which skin reaction would *not* be associated with wearing gloves in the clinic?
    a. irritant contact dermatitis
    b. allergic contact dermatitis
    c. latex hypersensitivity
    d. chemical hypersensitivity

27. Which statement regarding clinical masks is correct?
    a. They protect against exposure to TB.
    b. They reduce the inhalation of dental aerosols.
    c. They prevent spatter from contacting mucous membranes.
    d. They protect patients against cross–contamination.

28. Bacterial filtration efficiency is a measure of effectiveness for which aspect of PPE?
    a. gloves
    b. masks
    c. protective eyewear
    d. protective clothing

29. When should one change protective clothing?
    a. after every patient
    b. each half-day of work
    c. when visibly soiled
    d. after using a high-speed handpiece

30. Removal of which item of PPE is required when temporarily leaving the operatory?
    a. protective clothing
    b. protective eyewear
    c. surgical mask
    d. gloves

31. What does a number "4" in the red-colored section of a hazard class sticker mean?
    a. The chemical poses a modest health hazard to workers.
    b. The chemical is normally unstable and can undergo rapid, violent change.
    c. The chemical is more expensive that other similar types.
    d. The chemical vaporizes quickly at room temperature and burns readily.

32. How should exposed dental film be transferred to an automatic processor?
    a. wrapped in a towel and placed in the pocket of a clinic jacket
    b. sealed in protective pouches
    c. carried in a gloved hand
    d. carried in a plastic cup

33. Which listed item is *not* considered to be a hazardous chemical?
    a. bleach
    b. ethyl alcohol
    c. aspirin
    d. amalgam

34. Who is responsible for designating a chemical as hazardous?
  a. employers
  b. the EPA
  c. employees
  d. manufacturers

35. Hazardous chemicals in the dental office should include which identifier?
  a. a matching MSDS
  b. a specific warning sign
  c. the amount present in the workplace
  d. flammability designation

36. In a dental office, countertops are classified as which type of surface?
  a. touch
  b. clinical
  c. spatter
  d. transfer

37. What is another name for the Hazard Communication Standard?
  a. chemical safety law
  b. employee training law
  c. employee right-to-know law
  d. hazardous waste law

38. Use of liquid sterilants, such as glutaraldehyde, is restricted to which type of reusable items?
  a. metal
  b. blood contaminated
  c. heat sensitive
  d. critical level

39. Which listed item is *not* considered to be a hazardous chemical?
  a. bleach
  b. ethyl alcohol
  c. aspirin
  d. amalgam

40. Which of the following statements is accurate as it refers to precleaning work surfaces in a dental office?
  a. Soap and water precleaning saves time over the use of a disinfectant that cleans as well as disinfects.
  b. If a surface is not clean, it cannot be disinfected.
  c. *Precleaning* and *disinfecting* are synonymous terms.
  d. Precleaning is only necessary if blood is present on the surface.

41. In a dental office, which mode of transmission of hepatitis B virus is most efficient?
  a. direct transmission
  b. indirect transmission
  c. droplet infection
  d. airborne infection

42. Which source of disease transmission is the most prevalent in dental offices?
  a. practitioner's hands
  b. airborne particles
  c. water
  d. patients' mouths

43. Which statement best defines the term *standard precautions*?
a. All patients are treated as though they are infected with a bloodborne pathogen.
b. The same infection control procedures should be used for all types of health care facilities.
c. All patient blood and body fluids are potentially infectious.
d. Use only infection control procedures formally approved by a government agency

44. Which mode of transmission will *not* spread HIV/AIDS?
a. sexual contact
b. mother to newborn
c. percutaneous
d. inhalation

45. Which factor is linked to emerging diseases?
a. caused by an unknown virus
b. occurs in children
c. was not previously recognized
d. is fatal in almost all cases

46. What is the risk of occupational acquisition of HIV/AIDS by dental assistants?
a. very high
b. high
c. modest
d. very low

47. Which type of hepatitis virus is *not* a bloodborne pathogen?
a. A
b. B
c. C
d. D

48. Which hepatitis virus has the longest incubation time?
a. A
b. B
c. D
d. E

49. Which hepatitis virus is most likely to cause infection after an exposure?
a. A
b. B
c. C
d. D

50. Which method produces the best protection against a hepatitis B infection?
a. engineering control
b. vaccination
c. work practice control
d. wearing gloves

51. Where would a person find a herpetic whitlow infection?
a. oral cavity
b. hands or fingers
c. eyes
d. genitals

52. Which mode of transmission is most common with tuberculosis?
    a. inhalation
    b. ingestion
    c. mucous membrane contact
    d. breaks in the skin

53. Which procedure is recommended when caring for a contaminated needle?
    a. steam under pressure with emulsion
    b. liquid chemical sterilants
    c. discard in sharps container
    d. discard in biohazard container

54. When is it appropriate to use an alcohol-based hand rub?
    a. a sink is available
    b. before another hand washing agent
    c. after another hand washing agent
    d. there is no visible soil on the hands

55. How long should one rub the hands together when washing with soap and water?
    a. 1 minute
    b. 2 minutes
    c. 3 minutes
    d. 4 minutes

56. Which procedure is recommended for cleaning medicament containers before storing them?
    a. steam under pressure with emulsion
    b. cold sterile solution for 1 hour
    c. cold sterile solution for 10 hours
    d. spray–wipe–spray with surface disinfectant

57. Which PPE items should be worn while cleaning contaminated instruments?
    a. heavy-duty utility gloves and protective clothing
    b. a mask, heavy-duty utility gloves, and protective eyewear and clothing
    c. a mask, examination gloves, and protective eyewear and clothing
    d. protective eyewear, a mask, and heavy-duty utility gloves

58. Which of the following can kill bacterial spores, tuberculosis, and viruses?
    a. low-level disinfectants
    b. intermediate-level disinfectants
    c. high-level disinfectants

59. What is the purpose of the Spaulding Classification System?
    a. ranks resistance of microorganisms to chemical disinfectants
    b. ranks instruments as to their potential to cause infection
    c. ranks disinfectants as to their ability to kill tuberculosis
    d. ranks the reaction by health care workers to disinfectants

60. Which technique is *not* recommended for cleaning dental instruments?
    a. instrument washer
    b. hand scrubbing
    c. ultrasonic cleaner
    d. enzymatic presoak

61. How should one process an x-ray beam alignment device that cannot be autoclaved?
    a. Throw them away and get some that can be autoclaved.
    b. Enclose them using a plastic wrapping material.
    c. Soak them in a high-level disinfectant.
    d. Clean them carefully with soap and water.

62. Which procedure should one follow when using a daylight loader?
    a. Keep some disinfectant inside the loader to treat film packets.
    b. Only open the film packets after they are in the loader.
    c. Only open film packets inside of plastic pouches inside the loader.
    d. Insert only disinfected or unsoiled film packets.

63. At which level are hospital disinfectants categorized?
    a. high-level disinfectant
    b. intermediate-level disinfectant
    c. low-level disinfectant

64. Which statement best describes the goal of infection control?
    a. Reduce the number of microorganisms shared between people.
    b. Increase the human body's resistance to microorganisms.
    c. Decrease the virulence of all microorganisms.
    d. Sterilize all instruments used on patients.

65. Which item helps protect both a dental assistant and dental patient from contamination?
    a. protective eyewear
    b. clinic gloves
    c. cover gown
    d. utility gloves

66. Which item should be removed if a dental health care worker temporarily leaves the treatment room during patient care?
    a. surgical mask
    b. protective eyewear
    c. gloves
    d. protective clothing

67. How often should one replace the plastic cover placed over the light handles?
    a. after every patient
    b. at least every half workday
    c. when the cover becomes visibly soiled
    d. only when damage to cover has occurred

68. Which member of the dental team is responsible for the initial opportunity to break the cycle of disease transmission?
    a. dentist
    b. dental hygienist
    c. chairside assistant
    d. administrative assistant

69. At which step should the potential for disease transmission be halted?
    a. donning PPE
    b. reviewing the medical history
    c. removing PPE
    d. preventing cross-contamination

70. Which area of the dental office would be least susceptible to cross-contamination?
    a. reception desk
    b. dental chair
    c. lab area
    d. operatory counters

71. Which microorganism is highly resistant to heat and chemicals?
    a. yeasts
    b. viruses
    c. spores
    d. staphylococci

72. What does the term *CFU* mean?
    a. counts found undetermined
    b. colony-forming units
    c. coli-forming units
    d. counts first undertaken

73. After sterilization what is the shelf life of unwrapped instruments?
    a. 24 hours
    b. no shelf life
    c. 1 year
    d. 3 months

74. What is the leading cause of sterilization failure in dental offices?
    a. mechanical malfunction
    b. poorly constructed instruments
    c. human error
    d. selection of wrong type of sterilizer

75. Why should instruments be presoaked before cleaning?
    a. to kill microorganisms
    b. to reduce bioburden
    c. to make cleaning easier
    d. to minimize rusting

76. Why should instruments be cleaned before sterilization?
    a. to increase the chance of sterilizer success
    b. to reduce instrument rusting and dulling
    c. to kill any microorganisms present
    d. to minimize instrument damage

77. When using an ultrasonic cleaner, which procedure is correct?
    a. Routine cleaning takes about 60 seconds.
    b. Use a basket for loose instruments or a basket or rack for cassettes.
    c. Hand scrub instruments before placement in the ultrasonic cleaner.
    d. Use dishwashing detergents; they work and are cheaper.

78. What is the rationale for packaging instruments before sterilization?
    a. helps minimize instrument rusting and dulling
    b. reduces instrument damage from occurring
    c. maintains instrument sterility after processing
    d. helps in organizing instruments into functional groups

79. Which combination of factors will produce the greatest amount of instrument rusting and dulling?
    a. carbon steel instruments in a steam sterilizer
    b. stainless steel instruments in an unsaturated chemical vapor sterilizer
    c. carbon steel in a dry heat sterilizer
    d. stainless steel instruments in a steam sterilizer

80. Which sterilizer is best biologically monitored by *Bacillus atrophaeus (subtilis)* spores?
    a. dry heat sterilizers
    b. steam autoclaves
    c. unsaturated chemical vapor sterilizers

81. Which sterilizer has the highest operating temperature and longest cycle time?
    a. dry heat sterilizers
    b. steam autoclaves
    c. unsaturated chemical vapor sterilizers

82. According to the CDC, how often should an office biologically monitor the sterilizer?
    a. each load
    b. weekly
    c. monthly
    d. every 2 months

83. Recording the highest temperature reached during a sterilization cycle is an example of which method of monitoring?
    a. physical or mechanical
    b. chemical
    c. biological

84. How often should one use chemical monitors in the sterilizer?
    a. with every instrument pack
    b. with one pack per load
    c. daily
    d. weekly

85. Why is it important to dry instrument packages inside the sterilizer after the end of a sterilization cycle?
   a. prevents wicking of microbes through wet packaging
   b. prevents instruments from sticking to each other
   c. prevents water spots from forming on instruments
   d. allows chemical indicators to work properly

86. What is the maximum acceptable level of bacteria in dental unit water as recommended by the CDC?
   a. 700 CFU/mL
   b. 900 CFU/mL
   c. 500 CFU/mL
   d. 400 CFU/mL

87. How would one define the term *potable water*?
   a. sterile water
   b. dental unit water
   c. drinking water
   d. chlorinated water

88. Instruments should be packaged for sterilization to:
   a. maintain sterility
   b. label and identify
   c. improve organization
   d. organize preset trays

89. What should one do before changing a vacuum line trap?
   a. No preparation is necessary.
   b. Remove and then heat sterilize the vacuum line.
   c. Flush bleach through the line and follow with a water flush.
   d. Evacuate a disinfectant–detergent into the line and flush with water.

90. Patient-to-patient cross-contamination may occur when a patient closes his or her lips around which of the following?
   a. air/water syringe tip
   b. saliva ejector tip
   c. high-volume evacuator tip
   d. metal prophylaxis angle

91. Which statement best describes the disadvantage of using disposable items?
   a. It does not always prevent patient-to-patient transfer of microorganisms.
   b. There is no need to process hard-to-sterilize items.
   c. Performance may be less efficient than their reusable counterparts.
   d. It may be more expensive than reusable types.

92. Which chemical used for disinfection is classified as a high-level disinfectant?
   a. sodium hypochlorite
   b. phenol
   c. iodophor
   d. chlorine dioxide

93. Which item is an example of regulated medical waste?
  a. used examination gloves
  b. disposable clinic gowns
  c. used anesthetic needles
  d. used masks

94. A sharps container is an example of which type of control?
  a. administrative
  b. work practice
  c. engineering
  d. personal

95. Which of the following is *not* a recognized type of regulated medical waste?
  a. extract teeth
  b. sharps
  c. used PPE
  d. liquid blood

96. Regulated medical waste comprises what percentage of a dental office's total waste?
  a. less than 5%
  b. 5%
  c. 6% to 10%
  d. greater than 10%

97. What should one do if the outside of a biohazard bag becomes contaminated?
  a. Process it through a steam autoclave.
  b. Disinfect the outside surface.
  c. Place it into the regular trash.
  d. Place it inside another biohazard bag.

98. How should a filled sharps container be sterilized before discarding?
  a. Process teeth with amalgam separately.
  b. Use the bagged cycle time.
  c. Process containers on their sides.
  d. Process containers with their vents open.

99. Hazardous chemicals in the dental office should include which identifier?
  a. a matching MSDS
  b. a specific warning sign
  c. the amount present in the workplace
  d. flammability designation

100. Which chemical agent is *not* recommended for use as a surface disinfectant in a dental office?
  a. iodophors
  b. chlorine-based products
  c. glutaraldehydes
  d. phenolics

Answer Keys and Rationales

TEST 2

General Chairside

1. In the Universal or Standard tooth numbering system, which letter represents the maxillary left primary second molar?
   b. The maxillary left primary second molar is tooth J in the universal numbering system. K is the mandibular left primary second molar. T is the mandibular right primary second molar, and C is the maxillary right primary canine.
   CAT: Collection of Data

2. Which classification of carious lesions form on the occlusal surfaces or the buccal and lingual grooves of posterior teeth?
   a. A CL I carious lesion includes the pit and fissures on the occlusal surfaces of posterior teeth and lingual pits of molars and the lingual pits of maxillary incisors.
   CAT: Collection of Data

3. The more fixed attachment of the muscle that is usually the end attached to the more rigid part of the skeleton is the:
   a. The origin of the muscle is the fixed attachment that is usually attached to the more rigid bone. The insertion attaches at the movable bone.
   CAT: Collection of Data

4. Which of the following teeth would *not* be found in the deciduous dentition?
   c. The primary dentition does not include the second premolar. It is a succedaneous tooth that replaces the primary second molar.
   CAT: Collection of Data

5. What does this charting symbol indicate?
   b. A single slash line across a charted tooth indicates that the tooth is to be extracted. After being completed, the slash is converted to an X. A symbol for the root

canal would be placed within the canal, and an impacted tooth is denoted with a red circle around the whole tooth, including the root.
   CAT: Collection of Data

6. What does this charting symbol indicate?
   a. Recurrent decay outlines the existing restoration in red to indicate decay in the area. A restoration charted in solid black indicates that the tooth has an existing amalgam restoration. An S is placed on the occlusal surface of a tooth to indicate a sealant in place, and an X is placed through the entire tooth to indicate a missing tooth.
   CAT: Collection of Data

7. On a cephalometric analysis, the abbreviation Na stands for:
   c. On a cephalometric analysis, the abbreviation Na stands for nasion.
   CAT: Collection of Data

8. If the charting conditions indicate that there is a furcation involvement, some type of symbol will be placed:
   c. Furcation involvement is charted in the furcation area of a multi-rooted tooth. A furcation is an involvement between two or more roots; therefore, a symbol would never be placed on the occlusal, apical, or cervical region to denote a furcation involvement.
   CAT: Collection of Data

9. What does this charting symbol indicate?
   a. A gold crown is indicated by outlining the crown of the tooth and placing diagonal lines in it. A SS is placed on a tooth with a stainless steel crown, a missing tooth is indicated by an X, and a post and core has a line drawn through the root to

indicate the post and follow the line into the gingival third of the crown, making a triangle shape in red to be completed in a different color when the area has been restored.

CAT: Collection of Data

10. What does this charting symbol indicate?
    b. A missing tooth is indicated by drawing an X through the tooth. A tooth to be extracted has a red diagonal line through the tooth or two parallel lines through the tooth. An impacted tooth has a red circle drawn around the whole tooth, including the root. A rotated tooth is indicated by an arrow curving in the direction of the rotation.

    CAT: Collection of Data

11. What does this charting symbol indicate?
    d. Veneers only cover the facial aspect of a tooth and are indicated by outlining the facial portion only. To chart a full crown, the crown of the tooth is outlined completely if it is porcelain; a diagonal line is all gold crown. A root canal is indicated by a line drawn through the center of each root. An implant is indicated with horizontal lines through the root or roots of the tooth. Red indicates the treatment is to be completed and black or blue that treatment is completed.

    CAT: Collection of Data

12. What does this charting symbol indicate?
    b. A fracture is indicated with a red zigzag line. An implant is indicated with horizontal lines through the root or roots of the tooth. Red indicates that the treatment is to be completed and black or blue that treatment is completed. A diastema is indicated when two red vertical lines are drawn between the areas where the space is visible. A root canal is indicated by a line drawn through the center of each root.

    CAT: Collection of Data

13. Which surgical procedure describes a hemisection?
    c. A hemisection is a procedure in which the root and crown are cut lengthwise and

removed. Removal of the apical portion of the root is an apicoectomy; the removal of diseased tissue through scraping is apical curettage; the removal of one or more roots without removing the crown is a root amputation.

CAT: Chairside Dental Procedures

14. How should a properly positioned dental assistant be seated?
    c. A dental assistant should be seated 4 to 6 inches above the operator to have better visibility to the oral cavity. A position lower or higher will not provide adequate access to the patient's oral cavity.

    CAT: Chairside Dental Procedures

15. Using Black's classification of cavities, in what class are caries along the cervical of a tooth?
    d. A class V carious lesion or restoration is found at the cervical third of the tooth. Class I are pit and fissure lesions on posterior teeth and lingual pits of maxillary incisors. Class II involves the proximal surface of premolars and molars. Class III involves proximal surfaces of incisors and canines.

    CAT: Chairside Dental Procedures

16. An ML restoration on tooth #9 is classified as a _____ restoration.
    c. An ML restoration on tooth #9 is a Class III restoration because it includes a proximal wall of an anterior tooth. Class I are pit and fissure lesions on posterior teeth and lingual pits of maxillary incisors. Class II involves the proximal surface of premolars and molars. Class V restorations are on the gingival third of the facial or lingual surfaces of a tooth.

    CAT: Chairside Dental Procedures

17. Which instrument is used to remove subgingival calculus?
    a. Subgingival calculus is removed using a curette scaler. Sickle and hoe scalers remove supragingival calculus. A sickle scaler is used to remove large amounts of deposits from supragingival surfaces. A chisel scaler is designed to break apart

bridges of supragingival calculus deposits between teeth, particularly in the anterior region. A hoe scaler is designed to remove ledges of calculus and heavy stain from the facial, lingual, and palatal surfaces of the teeth.

CAT: Chairside Dental Procedures

18. Forceps are used in this portion of the clamp while placing the rubber dam.

    b. The tips of the rubber dam forceps are placed in the holes to grasp the clamp and widen it to fit over the designated anchor tooth.

    CAT: Chairside Dental Procedures

19. Which classification of motion should the dentist and the dental assistant eliminate to increase productivity and decrease stress and body fatigue?

    d. Class IV and Class V motions should be eliminated. These motions waste time and place stress on the body, resulting in fatigue. Class I and II motions require the least amount or effort, and Class III motion requires moderate stress.

    CAT: Chairside Dental Procedures

20. Which is an accurate statement regarding the placement of an oral evacuator tip?

    d. The assistant should place the HVE tip first, and then the operator places the handpiece to enable the assistant to gain access to the site.

    CAT: Chairside Dental Procedures

21. If a left-handed operator is preparing tooth #14 for a crown, where does the dental assistant place the bevel of the high-velocity evacuator?

    c. A dental assistant would place the HVE tip parallel to the lingual surface of tooth #14 if the operator is left handed. If a right-handed operator were treating this patient, the assistant would place the tip on the buccal surface.

    CAT: Chairside Dental Procedures

22. Which of the following statements is *not* a concept of four-handed dentistry?

    d. A wide-winged chair back does not allow for the operator and assistant to sit

close enough to use proper four-handed technique, causing back pain and neck stress. All of the other answers are criteria for successful four-handed dentistry concepts.

CAT: Chairside Dental Procedures

23. Which type of handpiece can operate both forward and backward and can be used with a variety of attachments?

    b. The low-speed handpiece can operate both forward and backward and is able to hold a variety of angles and contra-angles for slow cutting, polishing, and abrading. These characteristics do not exist in most high-speed handpieces.

    CAT: Chairside Dental Procedures

24. When a Tofflemire matrix band retainer is used, which of the knobs or devices would be used to adjust the size of the loop of the matrix band to fit around the tooth and loosen the band for removal?

    d. The inner knob, D, adjusts the size or the loop of the matrix band to fit around the tooth and loosens the band for removal. A is the spindle pin, which holds the matrix band in the retainer, B is the diagonal slot that slides up and down on the spindle pin and helps to secure the band in place. The open slots are placed toward the gingiva. The outer knob tightens or loosens the matrix band in the retainer.

    CAT: Chairside Dental Procedures

25. What is the purpose of a barbed broach?

    b. A barbed broach is used at the beginning of an endodontic procedure to remove necrotic tissue from the canal. The sharp, barbed sides are only evident on the broach.

    CAT: Chairside Dental Procedures

26. Which instrument would be used to remove debris or granulation tissue from a surgical site?

    b. The surgical curette is designed with spoonlike working ends that enable it to be used to easily remove debris and granulation tissue from the surgical site. The rongeur forceps is used to trim

and remove excess alveolar bone after an extraction. The bone file smooths rough edges of the alveolar bone, and the periosteal elevator is used to cut periodontal ligaments to aid in tooth extraction.
CAT: **Chairside Dental Procedures**

27. Which of the following statements is *true* regarding the use of a universal matrix band and retainer?
    b. For ease of use, the operator places the matrix retainer on the buccal surface of the prepared tooth, and the wedge is placed from the lingual side at the proximal surface involved. To place the retainer in a different position would cause interference during placement of the restorative material. It is necessary to use a wedge with the Tofflemire to prevent overhangs in the restoration.
    CAT: **Chairside Dental Procedures**

28. A dental team is restoring an MOD preparation on tooth #4 with amalgam. Which item is *not* required to place this type of restoration?
    d. A Mylar matrix is used when restoring a tooth with composite resin. The wedges would be used with the Tofflemire retainer, the carver is used to carve the occlusal anatomy, and the enamel hatchet is used to smooth the walls of the proximal box during the preparation.
    CAT: **Chairside Dental Procedures**

29. An orthodontic positioner is designed to:
    b. An orthodontic positioner is a custom appliance that fits over the patient's dentition after orthodontic treatment to retain the teeth in their desired position and permit the alveolus to rebuild support around the teeth before the patient wears a retainer.
    CAT: **Chairside Dental Procedures**

30. Which of these instruments would *not* be a choice when placing gingival retraction cord?
    a. The explorer has sharp, pointed beaks that would not be conducive to the placement of gingival retraction cord. The other

instruments have blunt ends to aid in cord placement and not traumatize the tissue.
CAT: **Chairside Dental Procedures**

31. From the photograph, what is the procedure for which this tray would be used?
    b. This tray is assembled to assist in the delivery and cementation of a cast restoration. The bite stick, articulating paper, and Backhaus towel forceps all are clues to this set up.
    CAT: **Chairside Dental Procedures**

32. The instruments shown from left to right are:
    b. The photographs shown from left to right are the Howe pliers, wire-bending pliers, and ligature tying pliers. No bird beak pliers, posterior band remover, or ligature cutters are shown.
    CAT: **Chairside Dental Procedures**

33. Which of the following is *not* a postoperative instruction to control bleeding after a surgical procedure?
    d. Rinsing will cause bleeding to be accelerated and may cause a clot to become loose. Pressure should be used for at least 30 minutes, and strenuous work and physical activity should be restricted for 1 day.
    CAT: **Chairside Dental Procedures**

34. What is the endodontic test in which the dentist applies pressure to the mucosa above the apex of the root and notes any sensitivity or swelling?
    b. The palpation test is performed by applying pressure to the mucosa above the apex of the root and noting any sensitivity or swelling. The percussion test is performed by tapping on the tooth in question. Thermal sensitivity, or the cold test, is performed by isolating the tooth in question and applying a source of cold to determine a response. Electric pulp testers test a tooth's vitality with a small electric stimulus.
    CAT: **Chairside Dental Procedures**

35. The process by which the living jawbone naturally grows around an implanted dental supports is known as:
    c. An osseointegration is used to attach living healthy bone to a dental implant.

A subperiosteal implant is one with a metal frame that is placed under the periosteum but on top of the bone. A transosteal implant is an implant that places the metal framework surgically through the inferior border of the mandible. An ostectomy is a surgical procedure to remove bone.
CAT: Chairside Dental Procedures

36. The treatment used as an attempt to save the pulp and encourage the formation of dentin at the site of the injury is a(n):
    a. Pulp capping is the process of applying a dental material to a cavity preparation with an exposed or nearly exposed dental pulp in an attempt to encourage the formation of dentin at the injury site. The pulpectomy is the complete removal of vital pulp from a tooth and a pulpotomy is the removal of only the coronal portion of vital pulp from the tooth. An apicoectomy is the surgical removal of the apical portion of the tooth.
    CAT: Chairside Dental Procedures

37. The removal of the coronal portion of an exposed vital pulp is a(n):
    b. A pulpotomy is the removal of the coronal portion of a vital pulp from a tooth. This is a procedure indicated for vital primary teeth, teeth with deep carious lesions, and emergency situations. Pulpectomy is the complete removal of vital pulp from a tooth. An apicoectomy is the surgical removal of the apical portion of the tooth, and a root resection is the removal of one or more roots of the tooth.
    CAT: Chairside Dental Procedures

38. The instrument used to adapt and condense gutta-percha points into the canal during endodontic treatment is:
    b. A spreader or plugger is used in the canal to compact the gutta-percha points as they are placed. A Gates Glidden bur is used to enlarge the walls of the pulp chamber or can be used to open the canal orifice. An endodontic spoon has a longer shank than a traditional spoon excavator and is used to curet the inside of the tooth to the base of the pulp chamber. A broach is a barbed

instrument used to remove pulp tissue from the canal(s).
CAT: Chairside Dental Procedures

39. The surgical removal of diseased gingival tissues is called:
    b. Whereas gingivectomy the surgical removal of diseased gingival tissues, gingivoplasty is a surgical reshaping and contouring of these tissues. Whereas gingivoplasty is a surgical reshaping or contouring of the gingival tissues, osteoplasty is surgical contouring or reshaping of bone. An ostectomy is surgical removal of bone.
    CAT: Chairside Dental Procedures

40. A(n) _____ is a dentist with a license in the specialty of dentistry who provides restoration and replacement of natural teeth and supporting structures.
    d. A prosthodontist is a dentist with a license in the ADA-recognized specialty of dentistry that provides restoration and replacement of natural teeth and supporting structures. An endodontist is a dentist in the specialty that diagnoses and treats diseases of the dental pulp and periradicular tissues. A periodontist is a dentist with an advanced degree in the specialty involved with the diagnosis and treatment of disease of the supporting tissues. An orthodontist is a dentist who specializes in preventing, intercepting, and correcting skeletal and dental anomalies.
    CAT: Chairside Dental Procedures

41. Periodontal pocket depth is charted at _____ points on each tooth during a baseline charting procedure.
    c. Six points on the tooth are charted for periodontal depth in determining a baseline: mesiobuccal, buccal, distobuccal, distolingual, lingual, and mesiolingual.
    CAT: Chairside Dental Procedures

42. A periodontal pocket marker is similar in design to a _____.
    b. A periodontal pocket marker appears like cotton pliers but has beaks at right angles to enable marking to take place on the gingival tissue.
    CAT: Chairside Dental Procedures

43. A(n) _____ is an additive bone surgery that includes the reshaping and contouring of the bone.
    b. An osteoplasty is a surgical procedure in which bone is added, contoured, and reshaped. An ostectomy is a surgical procedure that involves the removal of bone. Gingivoplasty is a surgical reshaping or contouring of the gingival tissues. An apicoectomy is surgical removal of the apical portion of a tooth.
    CAT: Chairside Dental Procedures

44. From the instruments shown below, select the periosteal elevator.
    a. The periosteal elevator is a double-ended instrument with flat and sharp ends that enable the dentist to loosen the gingival tissue and to compress the alveolar bone surrounding the neck of the tooth. The other instruments from left to right are a luxating elevator, a surgical forceps, a surgical curette, and a surgical evacuator tip.
    CAT: Chairside Dental Procedures

45. Using Black's classification of cavities, a pit and fissure lesion on the occlusal surface of molars and premolars is considered a class _____ cavity.
    a. Class I lesions or restorations are found in the pit and fissure areas on the occlusal surface of molars and premolars. A class II lesion involves a mesial or distal surface of posterior teeth. A class III lesion involves the mesial or distal surfaces of incisors and canines, and a class V lesion occurs at the cervical third of a tooth.
    CAT: Chairside Dental Procedures

46. Which of the following instruments would be used to transport a temporary restorative material to a cavity preparation?
    d. A Woodson is a type of plastic instrument that is used to carry the temporary restorative material to the cavity preparation; it has a paddle and plugger end used to condense the restorative material. A Ward's C carver is used to carve amalgam in a smooth surface restoration. A #7 cleoid–discoid carver is used on the occlusal surface of an amalgam restoration to carve anatomic anatomy. An explorer has

a sharp, pointed tip that would not enable the temporary material to be condensed into the preparation.
    CAT: Chairside Dental Procedures

47. Which orthodontic pliers are used in fitting bands for fixed or removable appliances?
    b. Contouring pliers are used for fitting bands for fixed or removable appliances. Bird beak pliers are used in forming and bending wires; posterior band remover pliers remove bands without placing stress on the tooth. Howe pliers are used in placement and removal or creation of adjustment bends in the arch wire.
    CAT: Chairside Dental Procedures

48. Which of the following rotary instruments would cut fastest and most efficiently?
    c. A diamond stone is designed to provide maximum cutting capabilities. The diamond flecks on the tip of the instrument are some of the hardest materials available for bur design. The tungsten and stainless steel burs will more slowly cut tooth surfaces, but the green stone is used to smooth tooth surfaces.
    CAT: Chairside Dental Procedures

49. In selecting a shade for a composite restoration, under which of the following conditions should the shade be selected?
    c. The shade should be selected before tooth preparation and isolation and while the tooth is moist. Determine the shade if possible in daylight or with standard daylight lamps and not under ambient lighting.
    CAT: Chairside Dental Procedures

50. When cleaning a dental handpiece, it is important to:
    a. Each handpiece manufacturer has its own set of instructions related to cleaning and lubricating that should be followed.
    CAT: Chairside Dental Procedures

51. A(n) _____ procedure is performed to remove defects and to restore normal contours in the bone.
    c. Osseous surgery is the procedure performed to remove defects and to restore

normal contours to the bone. The other procedures all relate to soft tissue surgery.
CAT: Chairside Dental Procedures

52. Which of the following is *not* a measurement used in constructing a complete denture?

d. *Reversion* is not a term used in dentistry in relation to denture construction.
CAT: Chairside Dental Procedures

53. All of the following are types of restorations *except:*

b. The classes of restorations are class I, II, III, IV, V, and VI. There are no class Xs.
CAT: Chairside Dental Procedures

54. _____ sealants _____ require mixing as they cure when they are exposed to UV light.

d. Light-cured sealants do not require mixing as they cure when they are exposed to UV light, unlike chemically cured sealants, which require mixing in order for the material to cure.
CAT: Chairside Dental Procedures

55. When adjusting a crown after cementation, the dentist most likely would use a(n) _____.

c. A stone is commonly used to adjust the crown after cementation because it will gently reduce the surface that needs to be adjusted without damaging the restoration. The other burs would be used to cut tooth tissue.
CAT: Chairside Dental Procedures

56. The procedure performed to remove subgingival calculus and to remove necrotic tissue from the periodontal pocket is referred to as _____:

d. Gingival curettage is the procedure that involves scraping or cleaning the gingival lining of the pocket with a sharp curette to remove necrotic tissue from the pocket wall. Root planning is a procedure that smooths the surface of the root by removing abnormal cementum that is rough or infused with calculus. Prophylaxis is the preventive procedure to clean and polish the teeth. Coronal polishing is the technique used to remove plaque and stains from the coronal portions of the teeth.
CAT: Chairside Dental Procedures

57. Why would a dentist use an intraoral camera?

c. Intraoral cameras are useful for many procedures, including gaining visual access to difficult areas of the mouth. An extraoral camera would be used to take a picture of the patient for the dental record, and a hand mirror would be helpful in demonstrating proper oral hygiene and periodontal depth.
CAT: Chairside Dental Procedures

58. To minimize leakage, what would the operator do to the rubber dam around each isolated tooth?

a. By inverting the rubber dam, the operator can keep a drier work area that will reduce saliva contamination. Ligating the dam is done between the teeth at the proximal surfaces. A punch is used to make the holes in the dam for the teeth to be exposed, and seal could have several references, but a seal is accomplished when the dam is properly inverted.
CAT: Chairside Dental Procedures

59. What are the attachments used for support or retention of a three-unit bridge called?

b. The tooth, root, or implant used as the support of a bridge is known as an abutment.
CAT: Chairside Dental Procedures

60. Which portion of the bridge replaces the missing tooth?

a. A pontic is an artificial tooth that attaches to the abutments of a fixed bridge to maintain space.
CAT: Chairside Dental Procedures

61. Which instrument would be passed to the operator to smooth the interproximal box on a prepared MO amalgam?

c. The enamel hatchet is used to plane the walls of the interproximal box of a class II restoration. A gingival margin trimmer is used to place bevels on the mesial or distal cervical margins. An interproximal carver is commonly a Ward's carver. A spoon excavator is used to remove debris from the tooth or aid in removing temporary crowns, temporary cement, or a permanent crown during try ins.
CAT: Chairside Dental Procedures

62. Which of the following would be considered a contraindication for a patient receiving a fixed bridge?

 d. To maintain a fixed bridge, the patient must demonstrate good oral hygiene. The other answers may impact a person's health, but they are not directly related to the placement of a fixed bridge.

 CAT: Chairside Dental Procedures

63. The surgical removal of the apex of an endodontically treated tooth is what procedure?

 b. An apicoectomy is a surgical procedure that removes the apex of an endodontically treated tooth that shows residual pathology on a radiograph and causes the patient discomfort. A hemisection is the surgical separation of a multirooted tooth through the furcation area. An extraction is the removal of a tooth, and pulpotomy is the removal of the coronal portion of vital pulp from a tooth.

 CAT: Chairside Dental Procedures

64. What is the common name for the #110 pliers?

 b. A generic name of this instrument is Howe pliers, and it is commonly referred to as utility pliers. Contouring pliers are used to crimp and contour the marginal edge of a temporary or stainless steel crown. Weingart pliers are used to place and remove arch wires, and a band pusher is used to push orthodontic bands into place during the try in and cementing steps.

 CAT: Chairside Dental Procedures

65. Before surgery, a patient is explained the procedure and then signs an authorization for treatment. What is this process called?

 b. Informed consent occurs when the doctor explains the procedure to the patient in terms that the patient can understand. The patient then signs the form stating that he or she understands and approves the procedure. Implied consent is consent in which a patient's actions indicates consent for treatment. Authorization for treatment is the form a patient signs or can also refer to an insurance company authorizing specific treatment for a patient. A release of information is the process during which

information about a patient is released to another person or agency after the patient has given permission to do such.

 CAT: Chairside Dental Procedures

66. A patient who is said to be "tongue tied" would have what type of procedure?

 b. Ankyloglossia, also known as "tongue tied," is corrected by a surgical procedure known as a frenectomy. An osteotomy is the smoothing or recontouring of bone, and an ostectomy is the actual removal of bone. An alveoplasty is surgical shaping and smoothing of margins of the tooth socket after a tooth extraction.

 CAT: Chairside Dental Procedures

67. The water-to-powder ratio generally used for an adult maxillary impression is _____ measures of water and _____ scoops of powder.

 a. The powder-to-water ratio should be 1 scoop to each measure of powder. For an adult maxillary impression, 3 scoops of powder and 3 measures of water are needed to adequately fill the entire tray.

 CAT: Chairside Dental Materials (Preparation, Manipulation, and Application)

68. If using a self-cure composite resin system, what will occur if the containers are cross-contaminated?

 a. By placing the contents of one jar into the other jar, a chemical reaction will occur, causing the material to harden.

 CAT: Chairside Dental Materials (Preparation, Manipulation, and Application)

69. Which statement is incorrect regarding tooth conditioner?

 b. According to manufacturer's directions, the acid-etching agent is not rubbed vigorously on the surface.

 CAT: Chairside Dental Materials (Preparation, Manipulation, and Application)

70. Which of the following materials would *not* be used to take a final impression for the creation of a prosthetic device?

 c. Alginate hydrocolloid is not a material of choice for a final impression for which some form of prosthetic device is to be made. This impression material may be used for study

models but does not have the strength or accuracy of the other listed materials.
CAT: Chairside Dental Materials (Preparation, Manipulation, and Application)

71. A porcelain fused to a metal crown would be designed so the porcelain would always be on which surface?
    b. The porcelain would appear on the buccal or facial surface of a tooth that is to be covered with porcelain fused to metal for aesthetic reasons.
    CAT: Chairside Dental Materials (Preparation, Manipulation, and Application)

72. A glass ionomer material may be used for all of the following *except* a(n):
    d. Glass ionomer material does not have an obtundant or soothing characteristic.
    CAT: Chairside Dental Materials (Preparation, Manipulation, and Application)

73. If the room temperature and humidity are very low while mixing a final impression material, the setting time may be:
    b. A cool, dry environment will allow more working time when mixing a dental impression material; thus, the setting time is increased.
    CAT: Chairside Dental Materials (Preparation, Manipulation, and Application)

74. A porcelain fused to a metal crown is being seated. The assistant will mix the cement to a _____ or _____ consistency.
    d. When seating a porcelain fused to a metal crown, the cement to be mixed must be of a thin consistency, referred to as a *cementation consistency*. This consistency is also referred to as the *primary consistency* rather than secondary, which is a thicker, firmer material.
    CAT: Chairside Dental Materials (Preparation, Manipulation, and Application)

75. A posterior tooth with a deep preparation may require a base that is designed to prepare pulpal defense by functioning as a(n):
    c. To protect the pulp, the dental cement provides insulation to the tooth from temperature and other environmental factors.
    CAT: Chairside Dental Materials (Preparation, Manipulation, and Application)

76. IRM (intermediate restorative material) is used primarily for:
    b. A provisional restoration is a temporary restoration, and the IRM material functions only as a temporary restoration for a period of time before a permanent restoration can be placed on the tooth.
    CAT: Chairside Dental Materials (Preparation, Manipulation, and Application)

77. A patient has a fractured amalgam on 29DO. Time in the doctor's schedule does not permit placement of a permanent restoration. Which of the following statements is *correct* as to the type of dental cement and the consistency that would be used in this clinical situation?
    a. Because a permanent restoration will be placed at a later date, a temporary restoration will be placed at this appointment. The patient will be biting on this restoration during normal mastication, so it must be a firm, heavy material as in a secondary consistency.
    CAT: Chairside Dental Materials (Preparation, Manipulation, and Application)

78. A reproduction of an individual tooth on which a wax pattern may be constructed for a cast crown is a(n):
    a. The reproduction of an individual tooth is called a "die." Upon this single model, a wax pattern is constructed to make the image for the cast crown. From an impression taken of the prepared tooth or teeth, a model is made. The die is the individual tooth within the model.
    CAT: Lab Materials and Procedures

79. Which food can be compared to a reversible hydrocolloid?
    c. Ice cream is a reversible hydrocolloid. A change in temperature causes the material to transform from one physical state to another. When the ice cream is frozen, it is in the gel state. When left at room temperature, the ice cream melts and turns into a solid state. When returned to the freezer, the ice cream again becomes a gel.
    CAT: Lab Materials and Procedures

80. An alginate impression has been taken to prepare a set of diagnostic models. Which of the following statements is *false* as it relates to handling the impression? Alginate impressions _____.

    d. Alginate impressions may not be stored in 100% relative humidity because the impression will absorb the moisture fairly quickly and the physical dimension of the impression will change. This type of impression should be stored in a moist towel for only a short period of time.
    CAT: Lab Materials and Procedures

81. A broken removable denture prosthesis can be repaired:

    c. A broken removable denture prosthesis can be repaired in the office with cold-cured acrylics. The patient should be discouraged from home repair because there is often only one chance to correctly approximate the relationship between the broken pieces. After the patient has "melted" the acrylic and placed the denture pieces in an incorrect relationship, it is usually impossible to repair the denture properly, and a new denture must be fabricated.
    CAT: Lab Materials and Procedures

82. The removable denture prosthesis can be cleaned in the dental office by all of the methods listed below *except:*

    d. Any one of the first three techniques may be used to clean a removable denture prosthesis in the dental office. Immersion in an ultrasonic cleaner with a special denture solution is an excellent way to remove plaque and debris. Brushing with a denture brush is also effective for accessible areas. Some patients will form tenacious calculus on dentures, and this can be removed by the dental hygienist with hand scalers and curettes. It would not be an effective method to attempt to clean the denture prosthesis in the patient's mouth.
    CAT: Lab Materials and Procedures

83. A patient is seen early in the morning. The record indicates she has diabetes. She mentions she had not yet had breakfast but took all of her medications before the appointment. As the appointment progresses, it is noted that she is perspiring, seems not able to focus on conversation, and is increasingly anxious. These symptoms are an indication of:

    d. The patient is displaying symptoms of hypoglycemia, low blood glucose. Because it was noted that she missed breakfast but took her medications, she should be offered a concentrated form of carbohydrate, such as a sugar packet, cake icing, or concentrated orange juice.
    CAT: Prevention and Management of Emergencies

84. Which of the following statements is *not* true as it relates to a patient's respiration?

    d. Respirations are normally lower in count per minute than the pulse rate. For instance, the normal pulse rate is between 60 and 80 beats/min, and the respirations per minute are between 14 and 18.
    CAT: Prevention and Management of Emergencies

85. What is the respiration pattern for a patient in a state of tachypnea?

    b. The respiration pattern of a patient in a state of tachypnea is excessively short, rapid breaths.
    CAT: Prevention and Management of Emergencies

86. What is the respiration pattern for a patient who is hyperventilating?

    b. When a patient is hyperventilating, the respirations will be abnormally fast and short.
    CAT: Prevention and Management of Emergencies

87. In an emergency, the staff member should feel for the pulse of a conscious patient at which artery?

    c. A conscious patient showing signs of distress will have his or her pulse taken at the radial artery.
    CAT: Prevention and Management of Emergencies

88. If a patient displays symptoms of hyperglycemia and is conscious, what is the first thing you should ask the patient?

b. You must determine when the patient last ate and if insulin has been taken before proceeding with any treatment.
CAT: Prevention and Management of Emergencies

89. Which of the following are the recommended guidelines for cardiopulmonary resuscitation?
    d. The American Heart Association guidelines for CPR recommend that immediate activation of the emergency response system and starting chest compressions for any unresponsive adult victim with no breathing increases the effectiveness of CPR. Thus, CAB—chest compressions, airway, and breathing—are the steps to be taken in CPR.
    CAT: Prevention and Management of Emergencies

90. Which of the following conditions is *not* a potential medical contraindication to nitrous oxide?
    d. Nasal obstruction, emphysema, multiple sclerosis, and emotional instability impact the use of nitrous oxide. Age is not a contraindication of the use of this substance.
    CAT: Prevention and Management of Emergencies

91. What substance is added to a local anesthetic agent to slow down the intake of the agent and increase the duration of action?
    b. A vasoconstrictor is used to slow down the intake of the anesthetic agent and increase the duration of the action of the local anesthesia.
    CAT: Prevention and Management of Emergencies

92. The type of anesthesia achieved by injecting the anesthetic solution directly into the tissue at the site of the dental procedure is known as _____.
    c. Infiltration anesthesia is achieved by injecting the anesthetic solution directly into the tissue at the site of the dental procedure and is generally used on the maxillary teeth because of the porous nature of the alveolar cancellous bone. A nerve block occurs when local anesthetic is deposited close to a

main nerve trunk. Field block anesthesia is injection of anesthetic near a larger terminal nerve branch. The anterior palatine nerve block provides anesthesia in the posterior portion of the hard palate.
CAT: Prevention and Management of Emergencies

93. General anesthesia is most safely administered in a:
    c. General anesthesia is most safely administered in a hospital setting or another facility such as the office of an oral surgeon with the necessary equipment for administration and the management of emergencies.
    CAT: Prevention and Management of Emergencies

94. Which of the following refers to an allergic response that could threaten the patient's life?
    c. Anaphylaxis is an allergic response that causes the tongue and throat to swell and interferes with normal breathing. Anaphylaxis can be fatal if not quickly treated.
    CAT: Prevention and Management of Emergencies

95. How should the staff respond if a patient is having a grand mal seizure?
    c. If a patient is experiencing a grand mal seizure, the staff should activate EMS and move potential hazards away from the patient to prevent serious injury.
    CAT: Prevention and Management of Emergencies

96. In which situation is nitroglycerin placed under the tongue of a patient?
    b. Nitroglycerin is placed sublingually for a patient who is experiencing chest pain from angina.
    CAT: Prevention and Management of Emergencies

97. MyPlate is an outline of what to eat each day. The smallest segment of the plate concept represents which food source?
    c. Protein sources vary depending on the age and gender of each individual. Limiting protein intake as well as fat content is imperative for a healthy diet.
    CAT: Patient Education

98. How are foods that contain sugars or other carbohydrates that can be metabolized by bacteria in plaque categorized?

b. Cariogenic foods are those that contain sugars or other carbohydrates that can be metabolized by bacteria in plaque to cause dental decay.

CAT: **Patient Education**

99. Organic substances that occur in plant and animal tissues are _____, and essential elements that are needed in small amounts to maintain health and function are _____.

c. Vitamins are organic substances that occur in plant and animal tissues, and minerals are essential elements that are needed in small amounts to maintain health and function. Both are essential for good health and body function.

CAT: **Patient Education**

100. Dry mouth is also known as _____.

c. Xerostomia is dry mouth caused by the reduction of saliva.

CAT: **Patient Education**

101. _____ is more prominent in older adults who have experienced gingival recession.

b. Cervical caries is of concern for elderly persons, who often have gingival recession. Carious lesions on root surfaces form more quickly than do coronal caries because cementum on the root surface is softer than enamel or dentin.

CAT: **Patient Education**

102. Which factor would *not* contribute to xerostomia in a patient?

b. Diet has little or no impact on xerostomia. Various systemic diseases, medications, and age all can contribute to xerostomia in a patient.

CAT: **Patient Education**

103. Which of the following would *not* be suggested as an intervention for the prevention of dental caries?

d. Although saliva could be stimulated, chewing mints is not a suggested intervention for prevention of dental caries. Mints contain sugar, which adds

to the potential increase in dental caries. The other answers all can contribute to intervention for prevention of dental caries.

CAT: **Patient Education**

104. A caries risk assessment test is used to determine the _____.

a. A caries risk assessment test is used to determine the mutans streptococci and lactobacilli count in the saliva.

CAT: **Patient Education**

105. Inflammation of the supporting tissues of the teeth that begins with _____ can progress into the connective tissue and alveolar bone that supports the teeth and become _____.

c. A patient may develop gingivitis in the oral cavity, and without intervention of improved oral hygiene, necessary dental care, and changes in diet, this condition can progress into periodontitis.

CAT: **Patient Education**

106. A dietary food analysis includes a diary of everything a patient consumes for:

a. A dietary analysis is completed by a patient for everything he or she consumes within 24 hours. Some dentists may ask to have this completed over several days, but 24 hours is used as the basic format.

CAT: **Patient Education**

107. MyPlate is an outline of what to eat each day. Which of the following statements is *true* regarding MyPlate?

c. The MyPlate concept supports a version for individuals who choose a vegetarian lifestyle.

CAT: **Patient Education**

108. The patient's record indicates that the status of the gingiva is bulbous, flattened, punched out, and cratered. This statement describes the gingival _____:

b. *Bulbous, flattened, punched out,* and *cratered* are all terms that are used to describe gingival contour.

CAT: **Patient Education**

109. When transferring patient records from the office to another site, the administrative assistant must do all *except* which of the following?

c. Patient records are not sent in their entirety to another site. These records must remain in the office. Only information that is requested and for which consent is given may be transferred.
CAT: Office Operations

110. A new filing system for clinical charts is to be installed in the office. Which of the following filing systems would be most efficient?

a. Open files with colored filing labels using alpha and numeric codes are the most common and efficient method for paper records storage. The other systems require more time and motion to use.
CAT: Office Operations

111. If an administrative assistant chooses to transmit a transaction about a patient electronically, under which Act does this task fall?

c. The Health Insurance Portability and Accountability Act (HIPAA) of 1996 specifies federal regulations ensuring privacy regarding a patient's health care information.
CAT: Office Operations

112. A message about a serious illness or allergy should be noted in which manner on the clinical record?

b. To protect a patient's privacy, information about a serious illness or allergy must be placed inside the record in a discreet but obvious manner such as a small, brightly colored label.
CAT: Office Operations

113. The group responsible for establishing regulations that govern the practice of dentistry within a state is the:

d. The Board of Dentistry in each state is responsible for establishing regulations that govern the practice of dentistry within each state. The membership and appointment of the members of these boards may vary from state to state. The ADA is a national professional organization for dentists. DANB

is the national agency responsible for administering the certification examinations and issuing the credential for the Certified Dental Assistant. CODA is a commission that accredits dental, dental assisting, dental hygiene, and dental laboratory educational programs.
CAT: Office Operations

114. The act of doing something that a reasonably prudent person would not do or not doing something that a reasonably prudent person would do is:

c. Negligence is the performance of an act that a reasonably careful person under similar circumstances would not do or conversely, the failure to perform an act that a reasonable careful person would do under similar circumstances.
CAT: Office Operations

115. A clinical dental assistant is hired in the practice. The dentist indicates that this person is to place an intracoronal provisional restoration. The person knows how to perform the task but does not yet have the EFDA credential required to perform the specific intraoral task. What should the new employee do?

c. A clinical dental assistant should perform only tasks that are legally assigned by state law and for which he or she is appropriately educated. If requested to do otherwise, it is the assistant's responsibility to inform the dentist that he or she is not legally qualified to perform a specific task.
CAT: Office Operations

116. The Good Samaritan Law offers incentives for health care providers to provide medical assistance to injured persons without the fear of potential litigation *except* under which of the following circumstances?

a. The Good Samaritan law was considered necessary to create an incentive for health care providers to provide medical assistance to injured people in cases of automobile accidents or other disasters without the fear of potential litigation. The law is intended for individuals who do not seek compensation but rather are solely interested in providing care to injured

people in a caring, safe manner with no intent to do bodily harm.
CAT: Office Operations

117. The objectives of good appointment book management include all *except* which of the following?
d. A good appointment book management system provides maximum productivity, reduction of staff tension, a concern for patient needs, and minimum downtime.
CAT: Office Operations

118. In reference to appointment management, *prime time* refers to:
b. Prime time is the most requested time. This may vary from community to community. Most commonly, it is time after school or after work.
CAT: Office Operations

119. Which time of day is considered most appropriate when treating young children?
c. Early morning time is a good time to schedule a young child because they are more alert and refreshed at this time. Trying to schedule a child during playtime or naptime can be strenuous for the caregiver.
CAT: Office Operations

120. What type of supply is a curing light used in the treatment room?
b. A curing light is a nonexpendable item because it can be reused and is not very expensive, like a capital item of several thousands of dollars.
CAT: Office Operations

Radiation Health and Safety

1. What is the appearance of a bent film?
b. Film bending or creasing causes a thin, black line in the corner of the film. When softening a film for patient comfort, the film may be creased too much, causing the emulsion to crack. A film that has been placed in the mouth backward and exposed will have a herringbone pattern. A scratched film will appear to have white lines. Static electricity will cause thin, black, branching lines.
CAT: Expose and Evaluate: Evaluate

2. What is the correction for an image that is foreshortened?
c. Foreshortened images occur with excessive vertical angulation. To correct this error, decrease the vertical angulation. This error occurs more frequently in the bisecting angle technique. Incorrect horizontal angulation results in overlapped contacts, and too flat a vertical angulation will cause elongation. The patient chin position would not have modified the result.
CAT: Expose and Evaluate: Evaluate

3. What is the most common reason to see a completely clear film?
b. The image appears clear when the film is not exposed to x-radiation. Other reasons for a clear film include failure to turn on the x-ray machine, electrical failure, or malfunction of the x-ray machine.
CAT: Expose and Evaluate: Evaluate

4. Why is the use of a thyroid collar discouraged in panoramic radiography?
b. A thyroid collar is not recommended for panoramic imaging because it blocks part of the beam and obscures important diagnostic information.
CAT: Expose and Evaluate: Assessment and Preparation

5. Which radiographic technique provides the most accurate representation of the tooth and surrounding structures?
b. The American Academy of Oral and Maxillofacial Radiology recommends the use of the paralleling technique for periapical images. The paralleling technique produces a radiographic image without

dimensional distortion. The bite-wing view shows only the crowns of the teeth in both arches. The panoramic view provides a wide view of the upper and lower jaws but not as accurate a representation of the teeth and surrounding structures. The bisecting technique is an alternative technique for periapical images but should only be used in special circumstances when the mouth is very small or patients have a low or flat palatal vault.
CAT: Expose and Evaluate: Acquire

6. The silver halide crystals are found in what component of the x-ray film?
   c. The film emulsion is a homogeneous mixture of gelatin and silver halide crystals. The silver halide crystals are suspended and evenly distributed in the gelatin. The film base is transparent and has a slight blue tint that is used to emphasize contrast and enhance image quality. This base provides a stable support for the emulsion and also provides strength. The adhesive layer is made of adhesive material that covers both sides of the film base. The protective layer is a thin transparent coating placed over the emulsion.
   CAT: Expose and Evaluate: Acquire

7. All of the following can be found in the cathode except one. Which is the EXCEPTION?
   a. The molybdenum cup, tungsten filament, and negatively charged electrode are found in the cathode; the exception is the tungsten target.
   CAT: Radiation Safety for Patients and Operators

8. What is the penetrating x-ray beam that exits the tubehead?
   a. Types of x-radiation are described as primary, secondary, or scatter. Primary radiation is the penetrating x-ray beam that is produced at the target anode and exits the tubehead. Secondary radiation refers to the x-radiation that is created when the primary beam interacts with matter. Scatter radiation is a form of secondary radiation

that occurs when an x-ray beam has been deflected from its path through interaction with matter.
CAT: Radiation Safety for Patients and Operators

9. X-rays are produced at the:
   a. X-rays are produced at the positively charged anode. The anode is the positive electrode inside the dental x-ray tube and is the location where electrons are converted into x-ray photons.
   CAT: Radiation Safety for Patients and Operators

10. What process is occurring in this image?
    b. Physiologic resorption is shown in this image. This is a process that is seen with the normal shedding of primary teeth.
    CAT: Expose and Evaluate: Evaluate

11. What is the radiopaque restoration in this image?
    b. An amalgam restoration on the mandibular first molar that has an overhang at the mesial cervical surface is visible here as a radiopaque restoration.
    CAT: Expose and Evaluate: Evaluate

12. What landmark is indicated by the arrows?
    a. The coronoid process appears as a triangle-shaped opacity. It is a marked prominence of bone on the anterior ramus of the mandible. It does not appear on a mandibular periapical radiograph but does appear on the maxillary molar periapical image.
    CAT: Expose and Evaluate: Evaluate

13. What type of radiograph is preferred to evaluate for an incisal crown fracture?
    c. The periapical image is recommended for the evaluation of a crown fracture. The periapical image allows the evaluation of the proximity of the pulp chamber to the fracture. The other views do not provide as clear an image for this condition as does a periapical view.
    CAT: Expose and Evaluate: Assessment and Preparation

14. Which of the following steps should be followed when exposing a panoramic radiograph?

   d. The patient should be instructed to close the lips on the bite block and to swallow once and then raise the tongue to the roof of the mouth to maintain that position during the exposure. Failure to do this will result in a shadow on the image.

   CAT: Expose and Evaluate: Acquire

15. To expose bite-wing radiographs, which size or sizes of receptors are used?

   b. Receptor sizes for bite-wing radiography range from 0 to 3 and vary according to use, dentist preference, and the size of the patient.

   CAT: Expose and Evaluate: Assessment and Preparation

16. Which is NOT an accurate definition used in dental radiography?

   c. A right angle is formed by two lines perpendicular to each other or an angle at 90 degrees.

   CAT: Expose and Evaluate: Acquire

17. Optimum time and temperature for manual processing is _____.

   d. Optimum time and temperature for manual processing is 68 degrees Fahrenheit at 4½ minutes is optimum. The other times and temperatures are inaccurate.

   CAT: Expose and Evaluate: Acquire

18. Which component of the x-ray film packet should be recycled?

   b. Recycling programs are available for the lead foil inserts as they are not to be disposed of with regular trash. Throwing the lead foil away in the trash is not recommended because of the amount of lead entering the environment. The film becomes the x-ray. The other materials may be discarded as standard waste.

   CAT: Infection Control: Standard Precautions for Equipment

19. If films are left in the fixer solution for 9 minutes, approximately how much time is spent in the developer solution?

   d. Fixation time is approximately double the development time; therefore, the answer is 4.5 minutes. The fixation time is dependent on the time the films remain in the developer solution.

   CAT: Expose and Evaluate: Acquire

20. What is the purpose of a step wedge radiograph?

   c. The step wedge radiograph compares different densities of radiographs that are processed daily, thus checking the strength of the processing solutions. This is a critical quality control procedure used for dental film and processing solutions. This process does not relate to film speed, light leaks, or the settings on the exposure panel.

   CAT: Expose and Evaluate: Acquire

21. When mounting a full mouth series, it is recommended to begin with which films?

   a. It is highly suggested and recommended to begin mounting a full mouth series with the bite-wing films. The bite-wing images give information to the dental professional regarding the maxillary and mandibular teeth on one film, thus aiding in the mounting procedure.

   CAT: Expose and Evaluate: Patient Management

22. Which statements are true about the lead apron?

   d. A lead apron should not be folded for storage purposes. When a lead apron is folded, it causes the lead in the apron to crack, thus leaving the patient susceptible to exposure. By storing the apron hanging on a rack, it preserves the longevity of the lead apron.

   CAT: Radiation Safety for Patients and Operators

23. Which cell would be considered to have high radiation sensitivity?

   d. The small lymphocyte has a high sensitivity to x-radiation because of its high mitotic activity and cell metabolism. The liver, nerves, and salivary glands are more radio-resistant and have lower sensitivity.

   CAT: Radiation Safety for Patients and Operators

24. When a radiographer is producing a radiographic image on a patient, it is recommended that the radiographer stand in which direction from the primary beam?
    c. Radiation health and safety guidelines require that the dental professional exposing a radiograph on a patient must stand 6 feet at a diagonal or perpendicular distance to ensure beam avoidance.
    CAT: Radiation Safety for Patients and Operators

25. What is the maximum permissible dose an occupationally exposed pregnant individual is allowed to accumulate in a year?
    b. The maximum dose equivalent that a body is permitted to receive in a specific period of time (occupationally exposed pregnant women) is 0.1 rem/year.
    CAT: Radiation Safety for Patients and Operators

26. If a radiographer cannot stand 6 feet away from the primary beam, which of the following should he or she do?
    b. Standing behind a lead-lined wall provides the radiographer with the necessary protection required to ensure that he or she is not being exposed to more than 5.0 rem in a year.
    CAT: Radiation Safety for Patients and Operators

27. When the dental assistant becomes the patient, where is the radiation-monitoring badge placed?
    d. Radiation-monitoring badges must be removed when the operator is having dental radiographs exposed because the badge measures occupational exposure only. The badge must be stored in a radiation-safe area.
    CAT: Radiation Safety for Patients and Operators

28. Which of the following relates to patient safety?
    d. The paralleling technique is a patient safety measure. All of the other answers relate to operator protection.
    CAT: Radiation Safety for Patients and Operators

29. Which of the following is a safety concern for the operator?
    c. Somatic effects could occur in the operator if there were any scatter radiation or leakage problems with the machine. The filter, thyroid collar, and thermionic transmission are all for patient protection.
    CAT: Radiation Safety for Patients and Operators

30. Which radiographic exposure is the best choice for the intraoral examination of large areas of the upper or lower jaw?
    a. A radiographic occlusal examination is used to inspect large areas of the maxilla or mandible on one image.
    CAT: Expose and Evaluate: Assessment and Preparation

31. When would tomography be used in dentistry?
    c. TMJ tomography provides the most definitive imaging of the TMJ's bony components. As a result, the condyle, articular eminence, and glenoid fossa can all be examined on a tomogram. This image can also be used to estimate joint space and evaluate the extent of movement of the condyle when the mouth is open.
    CAT: Expose and Evaluate: Assessment and Preparation

32. Which statement is NOT true about a bite-wing radiograph?
    c. The central ray of the x-ray beam is directed through the contacts of the teeth using a vertical angulation of 10 degrees.
    CAT: Expose and Evaluate: Assessment and Preparation

33. What will occur when voltage is increased?
    c. When voltage is increased, the speed of the electrons is increased. When the speed of the electrons is increased, the electrons strike the target with greater force and energy, resulting in a penetrating x-ray beam with a short wavelength.
    CAT: Radiation Safety for Patients and Operators

34. With faster F-speed film, a single intraoral film results in a surface skin exposure of _____ milliroentgens.
   c. With the development of F-speed film, the surface exposure, or the measure of the intensity of radiation on a patient's skin surface, has decreased significantly. Today, a single intraoral radiograph results in a mean surface exposure of 100 mR compared with the exposure of D-speed film a few years ago of 250 mR.
   CAT: Radiation Safety for Patients and Operators

35. Quality control tests that should be applied to dental office radiology standards should include which procedure?
   a. Providing regular maintenance on all equipment will keep it in good running condition and help discover issues that can be quickly resolved.
   CAT: Radiation Safety for Patients and Operators

36. In which exposure will the genial tubercle be seen?
   b. The genial tubercle and the lingual foramen are identified in the mandibular central exposure.
   CAT: Expose and Evaluate: Assessment and Preparation

37. What will occur if a lead apron is folded instead of hung?
   b. Lead aprons and thyroid collars must not be folded when stored. Folding eventually cracks the lead and allows radiation leakage.
   CAT: Radiation Safety for Patients and Operators

38. Which type of radiation byproduct is NOT associated with patient interaction?
   c. Tertiary is not a type of radiation interaction that would apply to patient exposure.
   CAT: Radiation Safety for Patients and Operators

39. Which type of lead apron should be used when exposing a panoramic radiograph?
   d. A double-sided lead apron is used for panoramic exposures to protect the front

and the back of the patient. A thyroid collar is not used because it blocks part of the beam and can obscure important diagnostic information.
   CAT: Radiation Safety for Patients and Operators

40. Which type of radiation is the penetrating x-ray beam that is produced at the target of the anode?
   c. Primary radiation is the penetrating x-ray beam that is produced at the target of the anode and then exits the tubehead. Other terms for primary radiation are *primary beam* and *useful beam*.
   CAT: Radiation Safety for Patients and Operators

41. Which statement would NOT be a function of the Consumer-Patient Radiation Health and Safety Act?
   a. The Consumer-Patient Radiation Health and Safety Act is designed to establish guidelines for the use and maintenance of x-ray equipment, not to dictate the number or type of radiographs to be taken for each patient. This latter duty is the responsibility of the dentist.
   CAT: Radiation Safety for Patients and Operators

42. Which term best describes the concept of radiation protection as it pertains to technique, amount, and quality?
   a. ALARA is a concept of radiation protection that states that all exposure to radiation must be kept to a minimum or "as low as reasonably achievable."
   CAT: Radiation Safety for Patients and Operators

43. The lack of which of the following actions could constitute patient negligence?
   a. Examples of negligent acts that could occur in a dental office include but are not limited to failure to obtain informed consent.
   CAT: Expose and Evaluate: Patient Management

44. What is the best way to limit a patient's radiation exposure?
   a. The first important step in limiting the patient's radiation exposure is the

proper prescribing, or ordering of dental radiographs. Using the fastest film, completing the exposures with no errors, and the use of a lead apron for the patient will all protect the patient but occur only after the initial order to expose the radiographs.

CAT: Radiation Safety for Patients and Operators

45. Under which situation is it NOT necessary for the patient to wear a thyroid collar?
    d. The only exception to the use of the thyroid collar is during extraoral exposures because it obscures information and results in a non-diagnostic image.

    CAT: Radiation Safety for Patients and Operators

46. What is the maximum permissible dose radiation for occupationally exposed workers?
    b. Radiation protection standards dictate the maximum dose of radiation that an individual can receive. The maximum permissible dose (MPD) for occupationally exposed persons who work with radiation is 5.0 rem/yr.

    CAT: Radiation Safety for Patients and Operators

47. What is a practical alternative for operator safety in the absence of a lead wall?
    b. The operator should stand at a 90-degree angle and at least 6 feet away from the tubehead.

    CAT: Radiation Safety for Patients and Operators

48. Which agency regulates the manufacture and installation of dental x-ray equipment?
    d. All x-ray machines must meet specific federal guidelines regulating diagnostic equipment performance standards. State and local governments may regulate how dental x-ray equipment is used and dictate codes that pertain to the use of x-radiation. Dependent on the local and state safety codes, dental equipment must be inspected and monitored routinely.

    CAT: Radiation Safety for Patients and Operators

49. Which factor is used to measure the penetrating power of radiation?
    b. Wavelength, the distance from the top of one wave to the top of the next wave, is used to measure the penetrating power of radiation.

    CAT: Radiation Safety for Patients and Operators

50. Which body tissue listed is the least sensitive to radiation exposure?
    c. The thyroid gland is the body tissue least sensitive to radiation exposure.

    CAT: Radiation Safety for Patients and Operators

51. What is the maximum permissible dose of radiation for a pregnant patient?
    a. The MPD of radiation for a pregnant patient should not exceed 0.8 rem/9 mo gestation period.

    CAT: Radiation Safety for Patients and Operators

52. Which situation could be used as an exception to placing the operator in the path of the primary beam?
    d. No matter what circumstances are present, a patient should always wear a lead apron with a thyroid collar when exposing radiographs.

    CAT: Radiation Safety for Patients and Operators

53. When x-ray exposure time is increased, there is _____ density of the radiograph.
    a. An increase in exposure time increases film density by increasing the total number of x-rays that reach the film surface.

    CAT: Radiation Safety for Patients and Operators

54. One reason patients object to having dental radiographs taken is_____
    _____.
    a. Scare tactics in public media and a lack of understanding of insurance benefits may cause a patient to ask a question regarding a radiographic procedure. The major reason for an objection to a radiographic or any other dental procedure is lack of education as to the value and or need.

    CAT: Expose and Evaluate: Patient Management

55. Misleading information as to the value of dental radiographs is from which of the following source?
   c. The source credited with misinformation is the popular press, not professional associations and professional journals.
   CAT: Expose and Evaluate: Patient Management

56. When asked by a patient about a dark area appearing at the root of a tooth, the response of the dental assistant should be which of the following?
   c. The dentist is legally licensed to diagnose dental problems. Diagnosis is not within scope of practice for the dental assistant.
   CAT: Expose and Evaluate: Patient Management

57. Proper chair adjustment for dental radiographs is which of the following?
   b. A patient should be in the upright position for a dental radiographic procedure. Reclining, even slightly, will alter the angle needed for a diagnostic outcome.
   CAT: Expose and Evaluate: Patient Management

58. Improperly stored film will appear _____.
   a. Improperly stored dental film will appear fogged. Light film is caused by underexposure; light bars at the edges are caused by a developing error; striped film is caused by a film placement error.
   CAT: Quality Assurance

59. Correct solution maintenance for manual film processing includes_____.
   a. Both developer and fixer need to be changed at the same time in a manual processor.
   CAT: Quality Assurance

60. _____results in deposits appearing on the walls of the processing tank.
   c. A reaction between the mineral salts in the water and carbonate in the processing process causes a precipitation on the walls of the processing tank. Contaminated solutions result in undiagnostic images.
   CAT: Quality Assurance

61. Dental x-ray film has the following properties EXCEPT: _____.
   d. Specific protocols are in place for storage, handing, and use of dental x-ray film. It does not, however, have a long shelf life. Boxes of dental film are dated, and storage protocols need to be in place to ensure film freshness.
   CAT: Quality Assurance

62. Optimal humidity in an area storing dental film is: _____.
   b. Dental film should not be stored in humidity below 30% or above 50%.
   CAT: Quality Assurance

63. A breakdown of chemicals in the processing solution that results from air exposure is the definition of which of the following terms?
   d. The breakdown of processing solutions is referred to as oxidation. Contamination occurs when one of the chemicals co-mingles with another; reduction of volume occurs with use; and exhaustion occurs when all the chemical energy is depleted from use.
   CAT: Quality Assurance

64. Of the following, which is added to the processing solution to compensate for oxidation?
   c. A preservative is used to counteract oxidation that occurs in the processing of dental radiographs. An acidifier is used in fixer solution to neutralize the alkaline developer. A hardener is found in fixer to harden and shrink the gelatin in the film emulsion after it has been softened by the accelerator in the developing solution. A restrainer is used to control the developer from developing the exposed and unexposed silver halide crystals.
   CAT: Quality Assurance

65. Rinsing dental film in the manual development process accomplishes which of the following?
   d. Rinsing developer solution from the film stops the development process. It is not done to change the fixing time. Film from the developer solution has not yet reached the fixer solution.
   CAT: Quality Assurance

66. A film that is exposed too closely to a safelight filter will appear _____.
 a. Fogging will occur when a film is processed too close to the safelight. A blurred image results from patient or tube head movement; films that appear too light or too dark are not the result of processing distance to the safelight.
 CAT: Quality Assurance

67. The film required for film duplication is called by which of the following terms?
 c. Creating an identical copy of a set of radiographs is called film duplication, and the film used is called *duplication film*.
 CAT: Radiology Regulations

68. Film duplication can be accomplished with the use of _____.
 c. Both manual and automatic processors can be used to make duplicate films, with equal quality.
 CAT: Radiology Regulations

69. It is best to retain dental records for at least _____ years.
 c. Dental records and dental radiographs should be retained for at least 7 years, with some variation depending on state laws. Ideally, they should be retained indefinitely.
 CAT: Radiology Regulations

70. Used developer solution is considered _____.
 d. Used developer is considered nonhazardous waste and can be disposed of in the sanitary drain.
 CAT: Radiology Regulations

71. Fixer solution and rinse water can be discharged into sanitary drain systems when _____.
 c. The only time fixer solution can be discharged down the sanitary drain is when all the silver halide crystals have been removed.
 CAT: Radiology Regulations

72. Undeveloped dental film must be disposed of in which of the following ways?
 d. Undeveloped dental film cannot be disposed of in normal office waste and must be collected by an approved waste management removal service.
 CAT: Radiology Regulations

73. Recycled radiographic material includes all of the following EXCEPT _____.
 c. Only the black wrapper of a dental x-ray film is considered not considered recyclable. Recovered silver from the fixer solution and lead foil can be recycled through appropriate vendors.
 CAT: Radiology Regulations

74. All employers must comply with OSHA Standards for Workplace Safety under which of the following conditions?
 d. There are no limiting circumstances; all employers must comply with the OSHA Standard for Workplace Safety.
 CAT: Radiology Regulations

75. OSHA guidelines must be adhered to by which of the following?
 d. OSHA guidelines apply to the entire dental healthcare team.
 CAT: Radiology Regulations

76. All Safety Data Sheets must be _____.
 a. All Safety Data Sheets, supplied by the manufacturer, must be kept on site.
 CAT: Radiology Regulations

77. Which type of material can transmit germs or certain diseases?
 b. An infectious material can transmit germs or certain diseases. Toxic materials are irritating to the skin, eyes, or lungs and can cause illness or death. Reactive materials can burn or explode when mixed with other materials such as air, water, or heat. Ignitable materials can ignite or burn easily.
 CAT: Radiology Regulations

78. Processing solutions are available in all EXCEPT which of the following forms?
 b. Processing solutions are available as a powder, ready-to-use liquid, and liquid concentrate but not vacuum-packed.
 CAT: Radiology Regulations

79. EPA-registered chemical germicides labeled as *hospital disinfectants* are classified as

    _____.

    c. EPA-registered chemical germicides labeled as *hospital disinfectants* are classified as low-level disinfectants. EPA-registered chemical germicides labeled as *tuberculocidal* are classified as intermediate-level disinfectants. EPA-registered chemical germicides labeled as *sterilants* are classified as high-level disinfectants.
    CAT: Infection Control: Standard Precautions for Equipment

80. Dental darkrooms should be disinfected with a/an _____.

    b. An intermediate-level disinfectant is appropriate for darkroom use.
    CAT: Infection Control: Standard Precautions for Equipment

81. Adjusting the chair and headrest, placing the lead apron, and removing metal objects from the head and neck area on a patient should be completed by the dental professional

    _____.

    a. Adjusting the chair and headrest, placing the lead apron, and removing metal objects from the head and neck area on a patient should be completed by the dental professional while he or she is not wearing gloves.
    CAT: Infection Control: Standard Precautions for Equipment

82. Films removed from the film packet that have not been in a barrier envelope are processed in a daylight loader with _____.

    c. Dental films that have not been protected by a barrier covering must be processed by an individual wearing a powder-free latex glove.
    CAT: Infection Control: Standard Precautions for Equipment

83. Which describes how a dental radiography film should be dispensed?

    c. Dental films should be dispensed in an envelope from a central dispensary.
    CAT: Infection Control: Standard Precautions for Equipment

84. Which best describes the function of a plastic barrier cover for a digital radiography sensor?

    d. A sensor will become contaminated with saliva, and the barrier serves as a protection.
    CAT: Infection Control: Standard Precautions for Equipment

85. After each use, before processing, each receptor must be _____.

    b. After each use, a receptor must be dried with a paper towel. Disinfection, barrier placement, or wiping with alcohol are inappropriate infection control measures.
    CAT: Infection Control: Standard Precautions for Equipment

86. Who determines the hazards of a chemical?

    b. OSHA determines the hazard of each chemical used in dentistry. The hazardous waste disposal service removes the waste according to local and state regulations. The employer follows the guidelines set by OSHA for the handing of a hazardous chemical, and OSAP helps close the gap between policy and practice.
    CAT: Infection Control: Standard Precautions for Equipment

87. Washing with a non-antimicrobial soap and water describes which term?

    c. Routine handwashing involves washing with a nonantimicrobial soap and water. Using an alcohol-based product would be termed an *antiseptic hand rub*.
    CAT: Infection Control: Standard Precautions for Patient and Operators

88. Which of the following statements regarding personal protective equipment (PPE) with radiography procedures is INCORRECT?

    a. PPE is worn by all dental professionals to prevent contact with potentially hazardous materials and is removed prior to leaving the dental office environment. However, PPE is NOT discarded after every patient contact.
    CAT: Infection Control: Standard Precautions for Patient and Operators

89. An instrument that does not contact mucous membranes is considered a _____ instrument.

    c. An instrument that does not contact mucous membranes is considered a noncritical instrument. An instrument that contacts mucous membranes and penetrates soft tissue or bone is considered a critical instrument. An instrument that contacts mucous membranes but does not penetrate soft tissue or bone is considered a semicritical instrument.
    CAT: Infection Control: Standard Precautions for Patient and Operators

90. Receptors collected from a series of radiographs must be placed in a receptacle bearing the patient's name. The operator should be _____.

    b. Receptors from a series should be placed in a cup by an operator with ungloved hands.
    CAT: Infection Control: Standard Precautions for Patient and Operators

91. Spatter of blood or saliva is not routinely associated with the exposure or processing of dental images.

    b. Although spatter of blood or saliva is not routinely associated with the exposure or processing of dental images, the transfer of infectious agents is still possible and universal precautions need to be applied.
    CAT: Infection Control: Standard Precautions for Patient and Operators

92. Which infection control practice in the dental health care setting applies to radiography procedures?

    b. Disinfection protocols are infection control practices in the dental healthcare setting that apply to radiography procedures. Vaccinations are not part of radiography procedure protocol, and PPE is not discarded after dental procedures. In addition, exposed film is not disinfected before it is developed.
    CAT: Infection Control: Standard Precautions for Patient and Operators

93. Which procedure must be prepared prior to seating the patient?

    e. Prior to seating the patient, image receptors and beam alignment devices are prepared.

    Removal of metal objects from the patient is done after the patient is seated.
    CAT: Infection Control: Standard Precautions for Patient and Operators

94. Which of the following occurs after glove removal?

    c. The lead apron is removed at the very end of the procedure with ungloved, uncontaminated hands. Transfer of contaminated equipment should be done with gloved hands.
    CAT: Infection Control: Standard Precautions for Patient and Operators

95. A commercially available plastic sleeve that fits over intraoral films is called a _____.

    a. A plastic sleeve used to cover intraoral films is called a *plastic barrier.*
    CAT: Infection Control: Standard Precautions for Patient and Operators

96. Which choice describes infection control protocol for an interrupted radiographic procedure?

    c. Gloves must be removed and hands washed prior to leaving a treatment area when an interruption occurs. The process is reversed upon returning.
    CAT: Infection Control: Standard Precautions for Patient and Operators

97. Which choice would be included in the benefits involved in the use of surface barriers?

    e. The use of barriers can reduce turnaround time and also the need for disinfectant. Surface barriers are not necessarily easy to apply.
    CAT: Infection Control: Standard Precautions for Patient and Operators

98. Which is the final step in handling film with barrier envelopes during processing?

    d. Once the films are exposed, they are dropped on a paper towel or into a container and then transported for developing; films are unwrapped and processed. The final step is to dispose of the barrier envelopes.
    CAT: Infection Control: Standard Precautions for Patient and Operators

99. Which of the following is the LEAST in concerns related to infection control in a radiographic procedure?

a. Microbes can be transferred directly, indirectly, or through aerosolization during a dental procedure. Water line biofilm contamination is least likely to occur during a dental radiographic procedure.

CAT: Infection Control: Standard Precautions for Patient and Operators

100. Which structure appears in this panoramic image?

c. The panoramic image in this question illustrates the metal framework for both maxillary and mandibular partial dentures with porcelain teeth in the posterior quadrants of both arches.

CAT: Expose and Evaluate: Evaluate

Infection Control

1. Which federal agency requires employers to inform employees of their risk regarding bloodborne pathogens?

b. OSHA mandates that employees know the risks associated with working with blood and receive training in bloodborne pathogens annually. The CDC is a nonregulatory federal agency that issues recommendations on health and safely. The FDA is a federal regulatory agency that is responsible for drugs, medical devices, animal feed, cosmetics, and radiation-emitting products. The EPA is a federal agency responsible for protecting and restoring the environment and public health through environmental laws.

CAT: Patient and Dental Healthcare Worker Education

2. According to OSHA, which type of control is responsible for reducing the risk of bloodborne pathogens in the workplace by confining or isolating infectious materials?

c. Engineering controls are measures designed to remove bloodborne pathogens and chemical hazards from the workplace. Administrative maintain records of activities, and work practice controls reduce the likelihood of exposure by alternating the manner in which tasks are performed. Housekeeping methods and procedures ensure clean and sanitary conditions in the workplace.

CAT: Patient and Dental Healthcare Worker Education

3. After initial training, how often should employees receive training concerning the OSHA Bloodborne Pathogens Standard?

c. In accordance with the OSHA Bloodborne Pathogens Standard, after initial training, employees must receive further training at least annually.

CAT: Patient and Dental Healthcare Worker Education

4. According to the Hazard Communication Standard, when should established employees receive training in hazard chemicals?

b. The Hazard Communication Standard requires training of an employee at the initial hiring and also upon the introduction of a new hazardous material or condition.

CAT: Patient and Dental Healthcare Worker Education

5. Which type of microorganism is the smallest?

b. Viruses are smaller than bacteria, ranging from 0.02 to 0.3 μm. Bacteria can range from 0.2 μm up to 1 μm wide and 5 to 10 μm up to 30 μm long.

CAT: Patient and Dental Healthcare Worker Education

6. What is the purpose of the Hazard Communication Standard?

b. The hazard communication program was developed to ensure that employers and employees are aware of work hazards and know how to protect themselves from potential injuries from hazardous materials. This program is not designed for patient or manufacturer use, although there may be an impact on each of these.

CAT: **Patient and Dental Healthcare Worker Education**

7. Who is responsible for providing MSDS?
   d. The manufacturer of the chemical product is responsible to provide an Material Safety Data Sheet (MSDS) for each product. An MSDS is a document that contains information on the potential hazards of a given product and how to work safely with the chemical product.

   CAT: **Patient and Dental Healthcare Worker Education**

8. With which hazards does section III of an MSDS deal?
   d. Section III of the MSDS provides information related to physical hazards associated with that particular material. Section II relates to hazardous ingredients, section IV discusses fire or explosive management, and section VI covers health hazards.

   CAT: **Patient and Dental Healthcare Worker Education**

9. Which factor contributes to the growth of biofilm in dental unit water lines?
   d. Water that is left standing in the dental unit water lines for a long period of time will accelerate the growth of biofilm. Biofilm can contain many types of bacteria, as well as fungi, algae, and protozoa.

   CAT: **Patient and Dental Healthcare Worker Education**

10. Which type of immunity is passed from mother to child in the womb?
    c. Natural passive immunity occurs when a mother passes antibodies to her child in the womb. Active immunity, also known as naturally acquired immunity, is generally long-term and can be acquired by a disease which a person contracted and then recovered. Artificially acquired immunity is obtained by vaccines in a process called immunization. Artificial passive immunity

involves the introduction of antibodies through means such as injection.

CAT: **Patient and Dental Healthcare Worker Education**

11. Which government agency requires employers to protect their employees from exposure to patient blood and other body fluids?
    d. OSHA's Bloodborne Pathogens Standard is the most important infection control law in dentistry for the protection of health care workers.

    CAT: **Occupational Safety**

12. Which government agency regulates the effectiveness of sterilizers?
    c. The purpose of the FDA is to ensure the safety and effectiveness of drugs and medical devices by requiring "good manufacturing practices" and reviewing the devices against associated labeling to ensure that claims can be supported. The other agencies do not regulate drugs and medical devices. The CDC is a nonregulatory agency that issues recommendations on health and safety. The EPA is a federal regulatory agency responsible to protect and restore the environment and public health through environmental laws. OSHA is a federal regulatory agency responsible to ensure the safety and health of workers by setting and enforcing standards.

    CAT: **Occupational Safety**

13. Which government agency regulates surface disinfectants?
    a. The EPA is associated with infection control by attempting to ensure the safety and effectiveness of disinfectants. Information on the safety and effectiveness of disinfectants must be submitted by manufacturers to the EPA for review to make sure that safety and antimicrobial claims stated for the products are supported by scientific evidence. The other agencies do not regulate the safety and effectiveness of disinfectants. The CDC is a nonregulatory agency that

issues recommendations on health and safety. OSHA is a federal regulatory agency responsible to ensure the safety and health of workers by setting and enforcing standards. The FDA is the agency responsible for safety and effectiveness of drugs and medical devices by requiring "good manufacturing practices" and reviewing the devices against associated labeling to ensure that claims can be supported

CAT: Occupational Safety

14. Biofilm in dental unit water lines could contaminate dental personnel through which method?

   a. Dental personnel could be contaminated by dental unit biofilm through aerosol spray. It is vital that all chairside workers wear personal protective equipment such as masks, gowns, gloves, and glasses during patient care.

   CAT: Occupational Safety

15. Which agency is dedicated to infection control in dentistry?

   c. The Organization for Safety and Asepsis Procedures, founded in 1984 and formally incorporated as a nonprofit organization in 1986, is considered the resource for dentistry for infection control and occupational safety and health. The Association for Advancement of Medical Instrumentation is an organization developed to support the health care community in the development, management, and use of safe and effective medical technology.

   CAT: Occupational Safety

16. Extracted teeth are considered what type of waste?

   b. Extracted teeth should be disposed of as regulated medical waste and should not be returned to the patient.

   CAT: Occupational Safety

17. When are opportunistic infections most likely to strike?

   a. An opportunistic infection will take advantage of an individual

who is in the recovery phase and the immune system is already compromised

CAT: Occupational Safety

18. How often should dental health care workers receive the influenza vaccine?

   c. For their own well-being and the health of their patients and families, dental health care workers should receive the influenza vaccine annually.

   CAT: Occupational Safety

19. Which method is *not* recommended for sterilizing handpieces?

   a. Handpieces should be sterilized by the method recommended by the manufacturer. Most handpieces can be processed by steam under pressure. The handpiece is first cleaned and lubricated according to manufacturer's directions, then packaged for storage and sterilized. Flash sterilizing is used for unpackaged instruments. Cold chemical and dry heat are not options for the handpiece since they first would cause chemical damage and dry heat would cause long exposure to the heat thus damaging the handpiece.

   CAT: Occupational Safety

20. How often should one receive the tetanus vaccine?

   d. The CDC Advisory Committee on Immunization Practices recommends that boosters need to be given only every 10 years.

   CAT: Occupational Safety

21. Who is responsible for paying the cost of vaccinating at-risk employees against hepatitis B?

   b. In accordance with the OSHA Bloodborne Pathogens Standard, hepatitis B vaccination performance standards states that employers must provide information on the vaccine, including the efficacy, safety, and method of administration, as well as the benefits of being vaccinated and the assurance that all medical records concerning

the vaccination process will be kept confidential. In addition, the vaccine is to be provided by employers and be given under the supervision of a physician.
CAT: Occupational Safety

22. For which illness is there currently no available vaccine?
    b. Vaccines do not exist for all diseases from which dental health care workers are exposed. Hepatitis C is one of the diseases for which there is currently no vaccine available.
    CAT: Occupational Safety

23. What is the last piece of personal protective equipment put on before treating a patient?
    d. Gloves are the last piece of personal protective equipment that should be put on before treating a patient.
    CAT: Occupational Safety

24. What is the first piece of personal protective equipment taken off after treating a patient?
    b. When removing personal barriers, the disposable gown would be removed first; it is pulled off over gloved hands, turning it inside out and immediately placing it into a waste receptacle. Avoid touching any underlying clothes when removing protective clothing.
    CAT: Occupational Safety

25. Which type of gloves should one wear when assisting during the placement of an amalgam?
    c. During routine patient care, the dental health care worker wears disposable latex or nonlatex examination gloves.
    CAT: Occupational Safety

26. Which skin reaction would *not* be associated with wearing gloves in the clinic?
    d. Chemical reactions would not be associated with causing a skin reaction from wearing gloves in the clinical setting.
    CAT: Occupational Safety

27. Which statement regarding clinical masks is correct?
    c. In dentistry, masks primarily protect the mucous membranes of the nose and mouth from aerosol sprays and spatter of

oral fluids from the patient or from items contaminated with patient fluids.
CAT: Occupational Safety

28. Bacterial filtration efficiency is a measure of effectiveness for which aspect of PPE?
    b. Face masks are composed of synthetic material that aids in filtering out at least 95% of small particles that directly contact the mask.
    CAT: Occupational Safety

29. When should one change protective clothing?
    c. When the outer clothing is obviously contaminated, it should be changed before providing care for another patient.
    CAT: Occupational Safety

30. Removal of which item of PPE is required when temporarily leaving the operatory?
    d. If a dental health care worker leaves the chairside during treatment, the gloves must be removed and a fresh pair placed before returning to chairside. An alternative is to place a pair of overgloves before leaving the chairside and removing these before returning.
    CAT: Occupational Safety

31. What does a number "4" in the red-colored section of a hazard class sticker mean?
    d. Red is the symbol identification code for flammability and indicates that the material will rapidly or spontaneously combust; blue is a health hazard; yellow is a reactivity hazard; and white is a special hazard, minimal hazard. The numbers 0 = minimal hazard, 1 = slight hazard, 2 = moderate hazard, 3 = serious hazard and 4 = severe hazard and indicates that the material will rapidly or spontaneously combust.
    CAT: Occupational Safety

32. How should exposed dental film be transferred to an automatic processor?
    d. After being wiped off with a disinfectant saturated wipe, contaminated films should be transported to the automatic processor by way of a small plastic cup or a plastic bag.
    CAT: Occupational Safety

33. Which listed item is *not* considered to be a hazardous chemical?
  c. Some chemicals are exempt from the HazCom Standard, including (but not limited to) aspirin.
  CAT: Occupational Safety

34. Who is responsible for designating a chemical as hazardous?
  b. The EPA is the agency that designates which chemicals are hazardous. This is not the responsibility of an employer or employee, and the manufacturer is responsible for providing the MSDS indicating the hazardous status of a chemical.
  CAT: Occupational Safety

35. Hazardous chemicals in the dental office should include which identifier?
  a. For each hazardous chemical product used in a dental office, there must be an MSDS on file.
  CAT: Occupational Safety

36. In a dental office, countertops are classified as which type of surface?
  c. The most common mode of cross contamination for countertops is from spatter. The next most common mode is touch.
  CAT: Occupational Safety

37. What is another name for the Hazard Communication Standard?
  c. The employee right-to-know law was established to ensure that all members of the dental team are aware and knowledgeable of the materials and hazards involved with their jobs.
  CAT: Occupational Safety

38. Use of liquid sterilants, such as glutaraldehyde, is restricted to which type of reusable items?
  c. Liquid sterilants are used for reusable items that cannot be heat sterilized. All other items should be sterilized by a heat sterilization system unless the manufacturer suggests otherwise.
  CAT: Occupational Safety

39. Which listed item is *not* considered to be a hazardous chemical?
  c. Some chemicals are exempt from the HazCom Standard, including (but not limited) to aspirin.
  CAT: Occupational Safety

40. Which of the following statements is accurate as it refers to precleaning work surfaces in a dental office?
  b. Precleaning reduces the number of microbes and removes blood, saliva, and other body fluids. If a surface is not clean, it cannot be disinfected. Soap and water may be used, but if a disinfectant that cleans as well as disinfects is used, time can be saved.
  CAT: Occupational Safety

41. In a dental office, which mode of transmission of hepatitis B virus is most efficient?
  b. The most efficient means of transmitting hepatitis B in a dental office is via indirect contact with items contaminated with the patient's microorganisms such as surfaces, hands, and contaminated sharps.
  CAT: Preventing Cross-Contamination and Disease Transmission

42. Which source of disease transmission is the most prevalent in dental offices?
  d. The major source of disease agents in the dental office is from the mouths of the patients. Microorganisms can be a source of contamination in other areas of the office, but by far patients' mouths present the greatest source.
  CAT: Preventing Cross-Contamination and Disease Transmission

43. Which statement best defines the term *standard precautions*?
  c. Standard precautions means to consider blood; all body fluids, including secretions and excretions (except sweat); nonintact skin; and mucous membranes as potentially infectious in all patients.
  CAT: Preventing Cross-Contamination and Disease Transmission

44. Which mode of transmission will *not* spread HIV/AIDS?

   d. HIV/AIDS is transmitted by intimate sexual contact, exposure to blood, blood-contaminated body fluids or blood products, and perinatal contact.

   CAT: Preventing Cross-Contamination and Disease Transmission

45. Which factor is linked to emerging diseases?

   c. Emerging diseases are new infectious diseases that until this time have not been recognized or are known infectious diseases with changing patterns.

   CAT: Preventing Cross-Contamination and Disease Transmission

46. What is the risk of occupational acquisition of HIV/AIDS by dental assistants?

   d. Studies of occupational risks of HIV infection for health care workers indicate the risk of occupational acquisition of HIV/AIDS is very low for this category of workers.

   CAT: Preventing Cross-Contamination and Disease Transmission

47. Which type of hepatitis virus is *not* a bloodborne pathogen?

   a. Hepatitis A does not pose an occupational risk for dental workers or patients because this form of hepatitis is spread primarily by the fecal–oral route involving consumption of contaminated food or water.

   CAT: Preventing Cross-Contamination and Disease Transmission

48. Which hepatitis virus has the longest incubation time?

   b. Hepatitis B has the longest incubation period of approximately from 6 weeks to 6 months. Hepatitis A's incubation period is from 2 to 6 weeks. Hepatitis D only affects those with hepatitis B and E, and the hepatitis is 15 to 65 days.

   CAT: Preventing Cross-Contamination and Disease Transmission

49. Which hepatitis virus is most likely to cause infection after an exposure?

   b. The evolution of the protective vaccine for hepatitis B is attributed to the decrease in the number of hepatitis B virus infections found in dental health care workers. The unvaccinated members of the dental team are at least two to five times more likely to become infected with hepatitis B virus than the general population.

   CAT: Preventing Cross-Contamination and Disease Transmission

50. Which method produces the best protection against a hepatitis B infection?

   b. Studies have shown a significant decrease in hepatitis B virus infections when a dental health care worker is vaccinated against this disease.

   CAT: Preventing Cross-Contamination and Disease Transmission

51. Where would a person find a herpetic whitlow infection?

   b. Herpetic whitlow is an infection of the fingers with herpes simplex virus. It is uncommon today because dental health care workers routinely wear gloves during treatment.

   CAT: Preventing Cross-Contamination and Disease Transmission

52. Which mode of transmission is most common with tuberculosis?

   a. The primary route of transmission is inhalation. Spread from one person to another relates to the closeness of contact and the duration of the exposure to infectious droplets.

   CAT: Preventing Cross-Contamination and Disease Transmission

53. Which procedure is recommended when caring for a contaminated needle?

   c. A contaminated needle is placed in the sharps container.

   CAT: Preventing Cross-Contamination and Disease Transmission

54. When is it appropriate to use an alcohol-based hand rub?

   d. When hands contain no visible soil, alcohol-based hand rubs without water and without rinsing have been shown to be effective in hand antisepsis.

   CAT: Preventing Cross-Contamination and Disease Transmission

55. How long should one rub the hands together when washing with soap and water?

a. The hands, nails, and forearms should be scrubbed using a liquid antimicrobial hand washing agent and soft brush for at least 1 minute.

CAT: **Preventing Cross-Contamination and Disease Transmission**

56. Which procedure is recommended for cleaning medicament containers before storing them?

d. Medicaments such as cavity liners or cement bottles can be disinfected using a spray–wipe–spray or wipe–discard–wipe to first clean and then disinfect the container before storing them.

CAT: **Preventing Cross-Contamination and Disease Transmission**

57. Which PPE items should be worn while cleaning contaminated instruments?

b. Utility gloves, protective eyewear, a mask, and protective clothing are all worn during instrument processing. These barriers provide personal protection from contaminants on the instruments and from the chemicals being used.

CAT: **Preventing Cross-Contamination and Disease Transmission**

58. Which of the following can kill bacterial spores, tuberculosis, and viruses?

c. According to the CDC, disinfectants are categorized according to their microbial spectrum of activity. High-level disinfectants destroy all microorganisms, including tuberculosis and viruses, but not necessarily high numbers of bacterial spores. Intermediate-level disinfectants are liquified disinfectants with EPA registration as a hospital disinfectant with tuberculocidal activity and are used for disinfecting operatory surfaces.

CAT: **Preventing Cross-Contamination and Disease Transmission**

59. What is the purpose of the Spaulding Classification System?

b. The CDC categorizes patient care items as critical, semicritical, and noncritical based on the potential risks of infection during use of the items. These categories are referred to as the Spaulding Classification System.

CAT: **Preventing Cross-Contamination and Disease Transmission**

60. Which technique is *not* recommended for cleaning dental instruments?

b. To protect the dental health care worker during instrument processing, protective utility gloves should be used, but instruments should not be scrubbed by hand. Instruments should be mechanically cleaned.

CAT: **Preventing Cross-Contamination and Disease Transmission**

61. How should one process an x-ray beam alignment device that cannot be autoclaved?

c. For maximum protection, beam alignment devices that cannot be autoclaved should be soaked in a high-level disinfectant. They cannot be thrown away nor enclosed in plastic wrap for normal use. Cleaning them carefully with soap and water does not meet the need for sterilization for this device.

CAT: **Maintaining Aseptic Conditions**

62. Which procedure should one follow when using a daylight loader?

d. to prevent cross-contamination, insert only disinfected or unsoiled film packs (those that have been placed in pouches) into the daylight loader. Operators should use powder-free gloves.

CAT: **Maintaining Aseptic Conditions**

63. At which level are hospital disinfectants categorized?

b. The EPA–registered hospital disinfectants are categorized as intermediate-level disinfectants.

CAT: **Maintaining Aseptic Conditions**

64. Which statement best describes the goal of infection control?

a. The goal of infection control is to reduce the number of microorganisms that may be shared between individuals or between individuals and contaminated surfaces.

CAT: **Maintaining Aseptic Conditions**

65. Which item helps protect both a dental assistant and dental patient from contamination?

   b. The use of gloves during treatment protects the dental assistant as well as the patients. Eyewear and a protective gown protect the assistant. Utility gloves are not worn at chairside but protect the assistant during instrument cleaning.

   CAT: Maintaining Aseptic Conditions

66. Which item should be removed if a dental health care worker temporarily leaves the treatment room during patient care?

   c. When a dental health care worker leaves the treatment room temporarily, the gloves must be removed and, when returning to chairside, the hands must be rewashed and regloved.

   CAT: Maintaining Aseptic Conditions

67. How often should one replace the plastic cover placed over the light handles?

   a. During treatment, these covers have been contaminated and must be changed after each patient.

   CAT: Maintaining Aseptic Conditions

68. Which member of the dental team is responsible for the initial opportunity to break the cycle of disease transmission?

   d. The administrative assistant provides the first line of defense by checking medical histories and reminding staff to remove contaminated PPE.

   CAT: Maintaining Aseptic Conditions

69. At which step should the potential for disease transmission be halted?

   b. Before the patient is called back for treatment, it is important to review the patient's medical history to look for potential issues that could lead to the transmission of disease.

   CAT: Maintaining Aseptic Conditions

70. Which area of the dental office would be least susceptible to cross-contamination?

   a. With the exception of a major break in infection control, the reception desk has least potential for cross-contamination.

   CAT: Maintaining Aseptic Conditions

71. Which microorganism is highly resistant to heat and chemicals?

   c. Some bacteria have developed a defense mechanism against death caused by adverse environmental conditions. A spore is a dense, thick-walled structure that enables a cell to withstand unfavorable environmental conditions. A spore or endospore is one of the most resistant forms of life against heat, drying, and chemicals.

   CAT: Instrument Processing

72. What does the term *CFU* mean?

   b. The term *CFU* refers to colony-forming units, or small groups of cells.

   CAT: Instrument Processing

73. After sterilization what is the shelf life of unwrapped instruments?

   b. Unwrapped sterile instruments have no shelf life and must be used immediately after sterilization.

   CAT: Instrument Processing

74. What is the leading cause of sterilization failure in dental offices?

   c. The primary cause of sterilization failure is human error; improper loading, improper timing, improper cleaning, improper packaging, and selecting the wrong sterilization method are all caused by human error.

   CAT: Instrument Processing

75. Why should instruments be presoaked before cleaning?

   c. Precleaning reduces the bioburden on the instrument and allows the sterilization method to be most efficient. A dirty instrument will not become sterile.

   CAT: Instrument Processing

76. Why should instruments be cleaned before sterilization?

   a. Cleaning instruments before sterilization will ensure proper sterilization. The FDA has approved ultrasonic cleaners and instrument washers for this purpose.

   CAT: Instrument Processing

77. When using an ultrasonic cleaner, which procedure is correct?
    b. Manufacturers of ultrasonic cleaners recommend using a basket for loose instruments or a basket or rack for cassettes.
    CAT: Instrument Processing

78. What is the rationale for packaging instruments before sterilization?
    b. Manufacturers of ultrasonic cleaners recommend using a basket for loose instruments or a basket or rack for cassettes.
    CAT: Instrument Processing

79. Which combination of factors will produce the greatest amount of instrument rusting and dulling?
    a. Carbon steel instruments placed in steam sterilization will promote rusting and dulling. This can be prevented by using distilled water in the sterilizer and a protective emulsion.
    CAT: Instrument Processing

80. Which sterilizer is best biologically monitored by *Bacillus atrophaeus (subtilis)* spores?
    a. To monitor a dry heat sterilizer, it is recommended that *Bacillus atrophaeus* strips be used.
    CAT: Instrument Processing

81. Which sterilizer has the highest operating temperature and longest cycle time?
    a. The dry heat sterilizer requires 60 to 120 minutes of processing at a temperature of 320° F.
    CAT: Instrument Processing

82. According to the CDC, how often should an office biologically monitor the sterilizer?
    b. The CDC, ADA, and OSAP, as well as the Association for the Advancement of Medical Instrumentation, recommend at least weekly spore testing of each sterilizer in the office. Some states require routine spore testing of dental office sterilizers.
    CAT: Instrument Processing

83. Recording the highest temperature reached during a sterilization cycle is an example of which method of monitoring?
    a. The personal monitoring or observation and recording of sterilizer activity are considered physical or mechanical monitoring.
    CAT: Instrument Processing

84. How often should one use chemical monitors in the sterilizer?
    a. Appropriate monitoring as recommended by the CDC involves the use of a chemical indicator on the inside and outside (if the internal indicator cannot be seen) of each pack, pouch, and cassette.
    CAT: Instrument Processing

85. Why is it important to dry instrument packages inside the sterilizer after the end of a sterilization cycle?
    a. Handling wet packages of instruments can cause them to tear and thus become contaminated. Exposing wet packages to the environment outside the sterilizer can cause wicking, a process that allows bacteria and fungi to penetrate wet sterilization paper.
    CAT: Instrument Processing

86. What is the maximum acceptable level of bacteria in dental unit water as recommended by the CDC?
    c. The EPA standard for the microbial quality of drinking or potable water is no more than a total of 500 CFU/mL (colony-forming units per milliliter).
    CAT: Asepsis Procedures

87. How would one define the term *potable water*?
    c. *Potable water* is the term used for water that is fit for consumption.
    CAT: Asepsis Procedures

88. Instruments should be packaged for sterilization to:
    a. Instrument packages should not be opened until the dental team is ready to use them. This practice ensures that the instruments maintain sterility before use.
    CAT: Asepsis Procedures

89. What should one do before changing a vacuum line trap?
    d. It is recommended that, before changing a vacuum line trap a detergent or detergent–disinfectant is evacuated through the system.
    CAT: Asepsis Procedures

90. Patient-to-patient cross-contamination may occur when a patient closes his or her lips around which of the following?

b. Research has shown that previously suctioned fluids might be retracted into the patient's mouth when a seal around the saliva ejector is created, causing a type of "suck back" or reverse flow in the vacuum line that might allow the contents to reach the patient's mouth.

CAT: Asepsis Procedures

91. Which statement best describes the disadvantage of using disposable items?

c. Disposables pose disadvantages, including the possibility of less efficient operation than the reusable counterpart, increased expense, and the addition of nonbiodegradable materials to the environment on disposal.

CAT: Asepsis Procedures

92. Which chemical used for disinfection is classified as a high-level disinfectant?

d. Chlorine dioxide is a high-level disinfectant that works in 3 minutes. It can also be used as a cold sterile agent when items are submersed for 6 hours.

CAT: Asepsis Procedures

93. Which item is an example of regulated medical waste?

c. Regulated waste is infectious medical waste that requires special handling, neutralization, and disposal. Used anesthetic needles fall into this category.

CAT: Asepsis Procedures

94. A sharps container is an example of which type of control?

c. Both engineering and work practice controls are used to minimize or eliminate exposure. In this example, a sharps container fits into the category of engineering controls.

CAT: Asepsis Procedures

95. Which of the following is *not* a recognized type of regulated medical waste?

c. Used PPEs are not a type of related medical waste. The other items listed all fall under regulated waste because they are potential infectious medical waste that require special handling and disposal.

CAT: Asepsis Procedures

96. Regulated medical waste comprises what percentage of a dental office's total waste?

a. Infectious waste is a small amount of the medical waste that has shown the capability of transmitting an infectious disease and comprises 3% or less.

CAT: Asepsis Procedures

97. What should one do if the outside of a biohazard bag becomes contaminated?

d. If the outside of a biohazard bag becomes contaminated, simply place it inside another biohazard bag.

CAT: Asepsis Procedures

98. How should a filled sharps container be sterilized before discarding?

d. In-house sterilization of filled sharps containers requires that the container must be autoclavable and that the container vents be left open.

CAT: Asepsis Procedures

99. Hazardous chemicals in the dental office should include which identifier?

a. For each hazardous chemical product used in the dental office, there must be an MSDS on file.

CAT: Asepsis Procedures

100. Which chemical agent is not recommended for use as a surface disinfectant in a dental office?

c. Of the agents listed, glutaraldehydes are not acceptable for use as a surface disinfectant in a dental office.

CAT: Asepsis Procedures

General Chairside, Radiation Health and Safety, and Infection Control

General Chairside

Directions: Select the response that best answers each of the following questions. Only one response is correct.

1. A patient displaying hypertension would have a blood pressure of about:
   a. 70/100 mm Hg
   b. 110/80 mm Hg
   c. 120/70 mm Hg
   d. 180/96 mm Hg

2. A patient presents appearing "flushed" and states that he has an infection. Which temperature would most likely be measured?
   a. 93°F
   b. 98.6°F
   c. 99.7°F
   d. 102°F

3. The normal blood pressure classification for adults is:
   a. 120/80 mm Hg
   b. 130/70 mm Hg
   c. 145/90 mm Hg
   d. 155/115 mm Hg

4. The most common site for taking a patient's pulse when performing cardiopulmonary resuscitation is the:
   a. radial artery
   b. carotid artery
   c. brachial artery
   d. femoral artery

5. Consent is:
   a. an involuntary act
   b. only necessary for surgical procedures
   c. something that any person older than age 21 years may give another's treatment
   d. voluntary acceptance or agreement to what is planned or done by another person

6. Using Black's classification of cavities, a pit lesion on the buccal of molars and premolars is considered a Class _____ restoration or cavity.
   a. I
   b. II
   c. V
   d. III

7. Any tooth that remains unerupted in the jaw beyond the time at which it should normally erupt is referred to as being:
   a. fused
   b. abraded
   c. impacted
   d. ankylosed

8. When assisting a right-handed operator, a preset tray is set up:
   a. left to right
   b. bottom to top
   c. top to bottom small to large
   d. right to left

9. The high-speed contra-angle handpiece reaches speed of:
   a. 150,000 rpm
   b. 250,000 rpm
   c. 350,000 rpm
   d. 450,000 rpm

10. An automated external defibrillator (AED) is used for all *except* to _____.
    a. reestablished the proper heart rhythm by defibrillation
    b. automatically perform CPR for 15 minutes
    c. monitor the patient's heart rhythm
    d. shock the heart

11. _____ can be life threatening and is indicated by nausea and vomiting, shortness of breath, and loss of consciousness.
    a. Syncope
    b. Anaphylaxis
    c. Low blood glucose
    d. High blood pressure

12. The respirations of a patient who is hyperventilating will be exemplified by:
    a. gurgling
    b. a slow respiration rate
    c. excessively short, rapid breaths
    d. excessively long, rapid breaths

13. The respiration pattern of a patient in a state of tachypnea has:
    a. a gurgling sound
    b. a slow respiration rate
    c. excessively short, rapid breaths
    d. excessively long, rapid breaths

Review the figure below to answer questions 14 to 18.

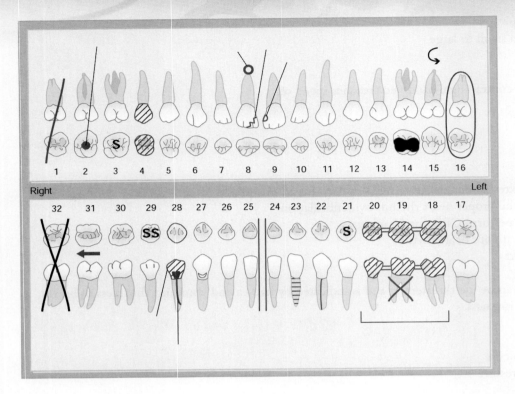

14. The symbol on tooth #31 indicates it is:
   a. mobile
   b. rotated
   c. drifted distally
   d. drifted mesially

15. The symbol on tooth #8 indicates it will need to have:
   a. periodontal treatment and then a restoration to replace the incisal edge
   b. endodontic treatment and then a restoration to replace the distoincisal angle
   c. periodontal treatment and then a restoration to replace the distoincisal angle
   d. endodontic treatment and then a restoration to replace the mesioincisal angle

16. The symbol between teeth #24 and #25 indicates:
   a. heavy calculus
   b. a diastema is present
   c. a supernumerary tooth is present
   d. a displaced frenum attachment

17. The symbol on tooth #23 indicates that this tooth:
   a. is an implant
   b. has a root canal
   c. has a post and core
   d. has a fractured root

18. The symbol on tooth #3 indicates that this tooth:
   a. has sealant placed
   b. has occlusal staining
   c. needs to have a sealant
   d. has a stainless steel crown

Review the figure below to answer questions 19 and 20.

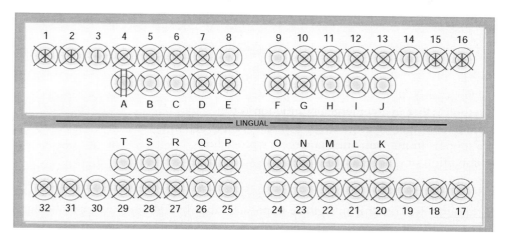

19. How many permanent teeth have erupted?
   a. 5
   b. 10
   c. 17
   d. 13

20. How many permanent teeth are present on the mandible?
   a. 6
   b. 8
   c. 13
   d. 15

21. The examination technique in which the examiner uses his or her fingers and hands to feel for the size, texture, and consistency of hard and soft tissue is called:
   a. probing
   b. palpation
   c. detection
   d. extraoral examination

22. A patient's pulse rate may be decreased because of:
   a. stress
   b. exercise
   c. stimulants
   d. depressants

23. Most local anesthetic agents used for dental procedures are:
   a. the same
   b. long acting
   c. short acting
   d. intermediate acting

24. In the United States, nitrous oxide gas lines are color coded, _____ and oxygen lines are color coded _____.
   a. red, blue
   b. green, blue
   c. blue, red
   d. blue, green

25. The dental assistant's responsibility in an emergency situation is to:
   a. recognize the symptoms and signs of a significant medical complaint
   b. provide appropriate support in implementing emergency procedures
   c. diagnose a specific condition or emergency situation
   d. both a and b

26. A condition called _____ will result if an alginate impression absorbs additional water by being stored in water or in a very wet paper towel.
   a. syneresis
   b. hydrocolloid
   c. imbibition
   d. polymerization

27. _____ may be applied to the edge of the alginate trays to improve the fit of the tray.
   a. Beading wax
   b. Pattern wax
   c. Utility wax
   d. Boxing wax

28. The water-to-powder ratio generally used for a mandibular impression is _____ measures of water, and _____ scoops of powder.
   a. 3, 3
   b. 4, 3
   c. 2, 4
   d. 2, 2

29. The term _____ means to move the tooth back and forth within the socket.
   a. festoon
   b. luxation
   c. capitation
   d. displace

30. _____ forceps are designed to grasp the bifurcation of the root of a mandibular molar.
   a. Curved
   b. Bayonet
   c. Cowhorn
   d. Universal

31. When a blood clot is dislodged because of the exertion of forces such as sucking on a straw and as a result the patient experiences extreme discomfort, it is referred to as:
    a. osteosis
    b. ankylosis
    c. alveolitis
    d. acidosis

32. The retromolar pad is reproduced in the _____ impression.
    a. maxillary
    b. mandibular

33. Which of the following instruments would be used to measure the depth of the gingival sulcus?
    a. shepherd's hook
    b. periodontal probe
    c. cowhorn explorer
    d. right angle explorer

34. Which of the following instruments has sharp, round, angular tips used to detect tooth anomalies?
    a. shepherd's hook
    b. periodontal probe
    c. cowhorn explorer
    d. right angle explorer

35. Which instrument is commonly used to scale surfaces in the anterior region of the mouth?
    a. curet scaler
    b. Gracey scaler
    c. straight sickle scaler
    d. modified sickle scaler

36. Which instrument is used to scale deep periodontal pockets or furcation areas?
    a. curet scaler
    b. Gracey scaler
    c. straight sickle scaler
    d. modified sickle scaler

37. In the drawing below, which area stabilizes the clamp to the tooth?

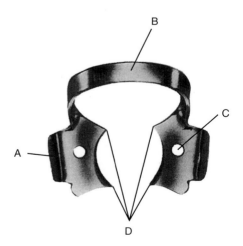

38. When the operator is working in the labial of tooth #9, the HVE tip is held:
    a. on the labial surface of the tooth being prepared
    b. on the opposite side of the tooth being prepared
    c. in the retromolar area
    d. in the vestibule

39. A right-handed dentist is doing a preparation on #30 MO. The dental assistant places the HVE tip:
    a. on the buccal of #30
    b. on the buccal of #19
    c. on the lingual of #30
    d. on the occlusal of #31

40. The angle of the bevel of the HVE top should always be:
    a. parallel to the occlusal surface
    b. parallel to the buccal or lingual surfaces
    c. at right angles to the buccal and lingual surfaces
    d. in whatever position the assistant is comfortable

41. The cement that has a sedative effect on the pulp is known as:
    a. glass ionomer
    b. zinc phosphate
    c. zinc oxide–eugenol
    d. zinc silicon phosphate

42. A wooden wedge is placed in the gingival embrasure area for Class II restorations to accomplish all *except* which of the following?
    a. aid in preventing overhangs
    b. adapt the band to the occlusal
    c. provide a missing proximal wall
    d. margin maintain proximal contact

43. Which of the following techniques could be used for caries removal?
    a. No. 2 RA bur and enamel hatchet
    b. No. ¼ FG and spoon excavator
    c. No. 2 RA bur and spoon excavator
    d. No. ¼ FG and explorer

44. Select the instrument that will be used to carve the distal surface of an amalgam restoration placed on 30DO.

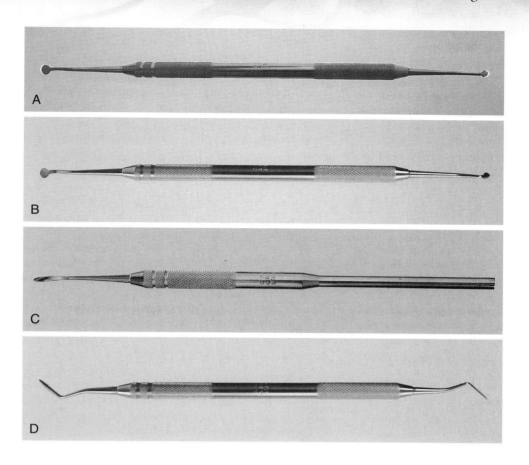

45. From the photograph below, select the instrument that would be used to attach to the rubber dam clamps.

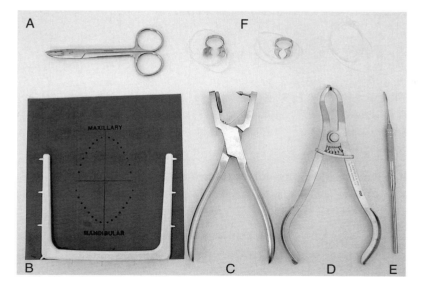

46. Which part of an anesthetic syringe differs in an aspirating and nonaspirating syringe?
   a. piston
   b. harpoon
   c. syringe barrel
   d. metal thumb ring

47. What is a contraindication for a patient using a gingival retraction cord that is impregnated with epinephrine?
   a. diabetes
   b. epilepsy
   c. hypothyroidism
   d. cardiovascular condition

48. Which instrument would be used to check for an overhang on a newly placed restoration?
   a. explorer
   b. Woodson
   c. spoon excavator
   d. Hollenback carver

49. Which of the following instruments would be the least likely to be used for placing a cavity liner?
   a. explorer
   b. ball burnisher
   c. spoon excavator
   d. amalgam condenser

50. Which of the following instruments is a Hedstrom file?

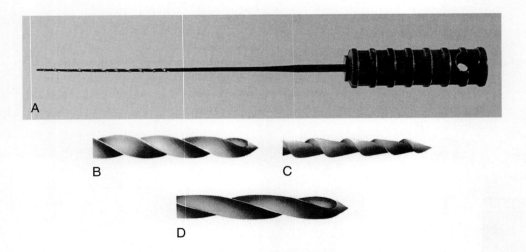

51. The purpose of acid etching a tooth when using a composite restorative is:
   a. preparing the pulp
   b. sealing the dentinal tubules
   c. forming tags on the etched tooth surface
   d. forming a bond on cavity structure of the tooth

52. Which of the following would be used for smoothing the interproximal surface in a composite procedure?
    a. Hollenback carver
    b. gold carving knife
    c. finishing strip
    d. explorer

53. Which endodontic instrument is used to curette the inside of the tooth to the base of the pulp chamber?
    a. file
    b. reamer
    c. explorer
    d. long-shank spoon

54. The indication for pit and fissure sealants is when teeth:
    a. are prone to caries
    b. are not prone to caries
    c. sealants are already present
    d. fossae are wide and easy to clean

55. A finger rest that stabilizes the hand to lessen possibility of slipping or traumatizing the tissue in the mouth is known as a _____.
    a. hinge point
    b. rest point
    c. fulcrum
    d. base

56. _____ is the form of anesthetic that renders the patient unconscious.
    a. Local
    b. General
    c. Inhalation
    d. Conscious sedation

57. A tooth that has been avulsed has been:
    a. fractured
    b. sealed with a sealant
    c. restored with amalgam
    d. knocked free from the oral cavity

58. The time from when the local anesthetic takes complete effect until the complete reversal of anesthesia is the _____ of the anesthetic agent.
    a. duration
    b. induction
    c. innervation
    d. compression

59. The lengths of the needles used in dentistry for local anesthesia administration are:
    a. ⅝ and 1 inch
    b. 1 and 1⅝ inches
    c. 1½ and 2 inches
    d. ½ and 1½ inches

60. The stage of anesthesia when the patient passes through excitement and becomes calm, feels no pain or sensation, and soon becomes unconscious is referred to as stage _____ of anesthesia.
   a. I
   b. II
   c. III
   d. IV

61. The most common type of attachment for fixed orthodontic appliances is the:
   a. orthodontic band
   b. bonded bracket
   c. arch wire
   d. separator

62. When a health contraindication is present that prevents the use of a vasoconstrictor, the retraction cord is impregnated with _____, and the cord may have a_____ agent applied to it to control bleeding.
   a. epinephrine, hemostatic
   b. aluminum chloride, galvanic
   c. sodium chloride, galvanic
   d. aluminum chloride, hemostatic

63. A(n) _____ is present when the maxillary teeth are positioned lingually to the mandibular teeth either unilaterally or bilaterally.
   a. overjet
   b. crossbite
   c. open bite
   d. end–to–end

64. What instrument is used in ligating an arch wire?
   a. hemostat
   b. Howe pliers
   c. ligature tying pliers
   d. utility pliers

65. A tray is set up from:
   a. left to right
   b. right to left
   c. top to bottom

66. A periodontal probe is an example of which type of instrument?
   a. examination
   b. hand cutting
   c. restorative
   d. accessory

67. Most local anesthetic agents used for dental procedures are:
   a. short acting
   b. intermediate acting
   c. long acting

68. At the correct therapeutic level, patients receiving nitrous oxide/analgesia will feel:
   a. slightly nauseated.
   b. the need to giggle.
   c. a floating sensation.
   d. anxious.

69. Which instrument is used for interdental cutting of gingiva and to remove tissue?
   a. Back-action hoe
   b. Orban knife
   c. Periodontal kidney-shaped knife
   d. Interdental file

70. Which of the following instruments is *not* included in the basic setup for most dental procedures?
   a. Curette scaler
   b. Mouth mirror
   c. Cotton forceps (pliers)
   d. Pigtail explorer

71. Which type of scaler has a rounded toe and rounded back and may be used supragingivally and subgingivally to remove fine calculus deposits?
   a. Sickle
   b. Hoe
   c. Universal curette
   d. Chisel

72. Which instrument is used to split or section a tooth for easier removal and to reshape and recontour alveolar bone?
   a. Rongeur
   b. Surgical chisel
   c. Bone file
   d. T-bar elevator

73. Which of the following instruments is used to trim soft tissue during an oral surgery procedure?
   a. surgical curette
   b. suture scissors
   c. surgical scissors
   d. scalpel

74. The HVE is used to keep the mouth free of saliva, blood, debris, and water; reduce bacterial aerosol spray caused by the high-speed handpiece; and_____.
   a. prevent dehydration of oral tissues
   b. help stabilize the patient's mouth
   c. retract the patient's tongue and cheek
   d. rinse the oral cavity during a procedure

75. When the high-speed handpiece is positioned on the occlusal surface of tooth #30, where would the assistant position the HVE?
   a. Buccal surface of tooth #30
   b. Buccal surface of tooth #29
   c. Lingual surface of tooth #28
   d. Lingual surface of tooth #30

76. Which of the following is true about the use of cotton rolls to isolate a working area?
   a. Difficult to apply
   b. Provide complete isolation
   c. Require frequent replacement because of saturation
   d. Rigid and inflexible for application

77. A wooden wedge may be used in which of the following class preparations?
   a. Tooth #31° cavity preparation
   b. Tooth #21^{OL} cavity preparation
   c. Tooth #15MO cavity preparation
   d. Tooth #3^{BO} cavity preparation

78. In an instrument tray setup, which instruments are placed farthest to the right?
   a. Hand cutting instruments
   b. Restorative instruments
   c. Additional examination instruments
   d. Basic setup instruments

79. Which of the photographs below illustrates an orthodontic hemostat?

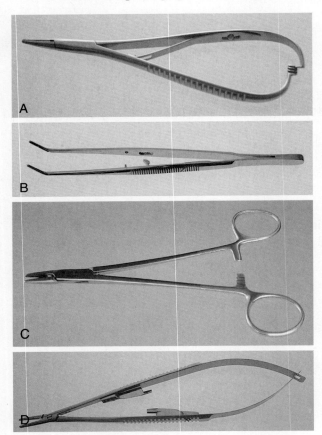

80. Which of the following is a thermoplastic material used to stabilize an anterior clamp?
   a. driangle
   b. floss
   c. dental compound
   d. sticky wax

81. Select two terms that describe the purpose and consistency of a dental cement used for the seating of a temporary crown.
   a. base and secondary consistency
   b. cementation and secondary consistency
   c. base and primary consistency
   d. cementation and primary consistency

82. Which type of cement must be mixed on a glass slab?
   a. zinc polycarboxylate
   b. zinc oxide–eugenol
   c. zinc phosphate
   d. calcium hydroxide

83. Which of the following materials is recommended for polishing filled hybrid composites and resin restorations?
   a. silex and tin oxide
   b. aluminum oxide paste
   c. diamond polishing paste
   d. coarse polishing paste

84. Light curing:
   a. relies on ultraviolet light.
   b. is used to polymerize composite resin restorative material and composite resin cement.
   c. is used to polymerize silver dental amalgam.
   d. is called autopolymerization.

85. The tip of the composite curing light should be held at an angle of __ degrees to the tooth.
   a. 10
   b. 25
   c. 45
   d. 90

86. Composite restorative materials are usually cured for __ seconds with a halogen curing light.
   a. 3
   b. 20
   c. 60
   d. 120

87. Hardness of a material is ranked using the:
   a. Richter scale
   b. Mercalli scale
   c. Moh scale
   d. atomic scale

88. Addition of very warm water to an alginate mix will cause the setting time to be:
   a. increased
   b. decreased

89. A negative reproduction of the patient's dental arch is referred to as a(n):
    a. die
    b. model
    c. cast
    d. impression

90. The impression automix system can be used for all but which of the following?
    a. syringe material
    b. tray material
    c. bite registration
    d. putty wash

91. The process by which the resin material is changed from a pliable state to a hardened restoration is known as:
    a. light curing
    b. exothermic curing
    c. microcuring
    d. macrocuring

92. The RDAs are the levels of essential nutrients that are needed by individuals on a daily basis. RDA stands for:
    a. recommended dietary allowance
    b. regulated daily amount
    c. regular daily amount
    d. recommended daily allowance

93. The only nutrients that can build and repair body tissues are:
    a. proteins
    b. fats
    c. carbohydrates
    d. minerals

94. _____ can prevent cholesterol from oxidizing and damaging arteries.
    a. Vitamins
    b. Minerals
    c. Lipids
    d. Antioxidants

95. A patient is to take a medication three times a day. The prescription will indicate to the pharmacy that it is taken:
    a. BID
    b. TID
    c. QID
    d. q.d.

96. If the signature line on a prescription states 1 tab QID prn pain, it indicates that the patient would take the medication:
    a. one tablet daily as needed
    b. one tablet every 4 hours for pain
    c. one tablet four times a day as needed for pain
    d. one tablet for 4 days

97. The eating disorder that can easily be recognized in the dental office by severe wear on the lingual surface of the teeth caused by stomach acid from repeated vomiting is:
   a. bulimia
   b. binge eating
   c. anorexia nervosa
   d. female athlete triathlon

98. Inflammation of the supporting tissues of the teeth that begins with _____ can progress into the connective tissue and alveolar bone that supports the teeth and become _____.
   a. gingivitis, glossitis
   b. periodontitis, gingivitis
   c. gingivitis, periodontitis
   d. gingivitis, gangrene

99. MyPyramid, formerly known as the Food Guide Pyramid, is an outline of what to eat each day. The food group represented by the second smallest section on the pyramid is:
   a. dairy
   b. meat and beans
   c. oils
   d. vegetables

100. _____ are found mainly in fruits, grains, and vegetables, and _____ are found in processed foods such as jelly, bread, crackers, and cookies.
   a. Proteins, carbohydrates
   b. Complex carbohydrates, fats
   c. Complex carbohydrates, simple sugars
   d. Proteins, simple sugars

101. Subgingival calculus occurs _____ the gingival margin and can be _____ in color because of subgingival bleeding.
   a. above, yellow
   b. below, yellow
   c. above, red
   d. below, black

102. The "A" in the ABCDs of basic life support stands for:
   a. access
   b. automatic
   c. airway
   d. assess

103. A patient who displays symptoms of intermittent blinking, mouth movements, a blank stare, and nonresponsiveness to surroundings may be displaying symptoms of:
   a. petit mal seizure
   b. grand mal seizure
   c. hypoglycemia
   d. hyperglycemia

104. In which of the following procedures could the patient be placed in an upright position?
   a. composite procedure
   b. removal of a posterior tooth
   c. polishing the teeth after a prophylaxis
   d. taking diagnostic impressions

105. Supragingival calculus is found on the _____ of the teeth above the margin of the _____.
   a. anatomic crowns, periodontal ligament
   b. cervical region, periodontal ligament
   c. clinical crowns, gingiva
   d. cervical margins, apex

106. Subgingival calculus occurs _____ the gingival margin and can be _____ in color because of subgingival bleeding.
   a. above, yellow
   b. below, yellow
   c. below, black
   d. above, red

107. The most common indication for placing pit and fissure sealants would include which of the following tooth characteristics?
   a. partially erupted teeth as a preventive measure
   b. posterior teeth with small areas of early caries
   c. all erupted permanent molars and premolars
   d. posterior teeth with deep pits and fissures

108. What step should the dental assistant take before applying topical fluoride?
   a. Give toothbrushing instructions.
   b. Have the patient rinse with mouthwash.
   c. Dry the teeth thoroughly.
   d. Use disclosing solution to look for plaque.

109. Which microorganism must be present for caries formation to begin?
   a. *Staphylococcus*
   b. herpes zoster
   c. *Candida albicans*
   d. *Streptococcus mutans*

110. Which energy nutrients come from plant sources?
   a. carbohydrates
   b. minerals
   c. proteins
   d. fats

111. A patient has the following amalgam restorations: 29MO, 30^{MOD}, 31DO, and 32°. The fee for each surface is $115. What is the fee for services rendered?
   a. $320
   b. $420
   c. $880
   d. $920

112. Consent is:
   a. an involuntary act
   b. voluntary acceptance or agreement to what is planned or done by another person
   c. only necessary for surgical procedures
   d. something that any person older than age 21 years may give for another's treatment

113. A dentist retires to another state and closes the practice. The entire staff is released from employment, and the records remain in the office, but the patients are not notified of the dentist's retirement. Failure to notify the patients of the changes in the practice is called:
    a. assault
    b. abandonment
    c. malpractice
    d. noncompliance

114. Which of the following is *not* a component of a clinical record?
    a. clinical chart
    b. health history
    c. medical history
    d. recall card

115. Which of the following records is considered a vital record?
    a. patient clinical chart
    b. bank reconciliation
    c. petty cash voucher
    d. cancelled check

116. Which member of the dental team is legally required to report suspected child abuse?
    a. all members
    b. dentist
    c. dental assistant
    d. dental hygienist

117. A dentist informs you that a patient will need three appointments to complete a three-unit bridge. These appointments will likely be to:
    a. prepare the teeth, try on the bridge components, and seat the bridge
    b. take diagnostic models, prepare the teeth, and seat the temporary or provisional crown
    c. prepare the teeth, take the impressions, and seat the bridge

118. An administrative assistant has failed to maintain the recall system for the past 4 months. Which is likely to occur?
    a. There will be evidence of decreased productivity.
    b. The patients will not mind.
    c. There will be more time to work on incomplete projects.

119. After a routine examination and prophylaxis of a 19-year-old female patient, the doctor diagnoses three restorations; the patient's mother calls to discuss her daughter's treatment plan. You politely and respectfully:
    a. proceed to review the treatment needed and answer her questions
    b. suggest she schedule an appointment for a consultation
    c. inform her that the practice must obtain consent from her daughter to discuss her care
    d. tell her that her daughter must be present during this conversation

120. A dental assistant orders supplies once per week and has been instructed to always maintain a 30-day supply of materials in the practice. The supply of syringes of composite shade A has been depleted and the practice uses these at a rate of one tube every 15 days. How many syringes should be ordered?
    a. one
    b. two
    c. three
    d. four

Radiation Health and Safety

Directions: Select the response that best answers each of the following questions. Only one response is correct.

1. Which of the following contribute to an underexposed image?
   a. The mA setting is too high.
   b. The kVp setting is too high.
   c. There is a light leak in the darkroom.
   d. Exposure time was too low.

2. Intensifying screens would be used with which of the following films?
   a. Bite-wing
   b. Occlusal
   c. Periapical
   d. Panoramic

3. Which is the true statement concerning the anode?
   a. It carries a negative charge.
   b. Electrons are generated at the anode.
   c. It consists of a tungsten filament in a focusing cup.
   d. It converts the bombarding electrons into x-ray photons.

4. During the production of x-rays, how much energy is lost as heat?
   a. 3%
   b. 10%
   c. 50%
   d. 99%

5. If the length of the PID is changed from 8 to 16 inches, how does this affect the intensity of the x-ray beam?
   a. The resultant beam will be one-half as intense.
   b. The resultant beam will be one-quarter as intense.
   c. The resultant beam will be two times as intense.
   d. The resultant beam will be four times as intense.

6. What is the effect on a film if the exposure time was decreased?
   a. The density increases; the film becomes lighter.
   b. The density increases; the film becomes darker.
   c. The density decreases; the film becomes lighter.
   d. The density decreases; the film becomes darker.

7. What is the type of contrast desirable when looking for periodontal disease?
   a. Low contrast; few shades of gray
   b. Low contrast; many shades of gray
   c. High contrast; few shades of gray
   d. High contrast; many shades of gray

8. What landmark is circled on the radiograph?
   a. Mental foramen
   b. Lingual foramen
   c. Mandibular canal
   d. Genial tubercles

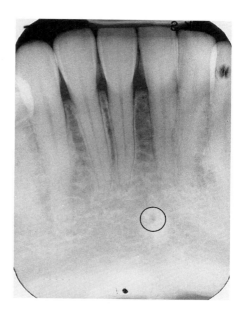

9. Which of the following pieces of equipment requires heat sterilization before use?
   a. Film
   b. Digital sensor
   c. X-ray tubehead
   d. Beam alignment devices

10. What landmark is indicated by the arrows?
   a. Zygomatic process of the maxilla
   b. Floor of the frontal sinus
   c. Floor of the maxillary sinus
   d. Zygomatic arch

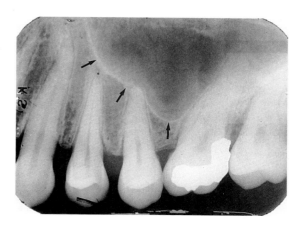

11. Which type of film is used in panoramic radiography?
a. Screen
b. Nonscreen
c. Duplicating
d. Intraoral

12. Which statement is NOT correct concerning the exposure sequence for periapical images?
a. Anterior images are always exposed before posterior films.
b. Either anterior or posterior images may be exposed first.
c. In posterior quadrants, the premolar image is always exposed before the molar image.
d. When exposing anterior images, work from the patient's right to left in the upper arch and then work from the left to right in the lower arch.

13. Which of the following conditions exists on this image?
a. A fixed bridge between the second premolar and second molar
b. Open contacts between maxillary premolars
c. Open contacts between the molars
d. Pulp stone on the second premolar

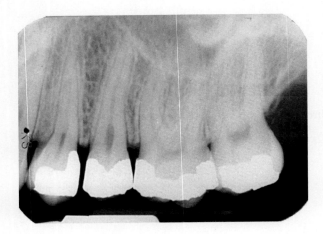

14. What is the appearance of the processing error termed "reticulation"?
a. Black film
b. Lighter film
c. Cracked emulsion
d. Yellow-brown stains

15. Label the solutions used in an automatic film processor from left to right.
   a. Water wash, developing solution, fixing solution
   b. Developing solution, fixing solution, water wash
   c. Fixing solution, developing solution, water wash

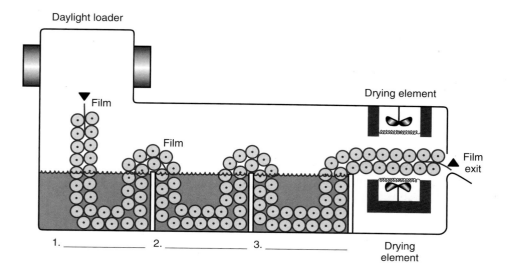

Daylight loader

Drying element

Film

Film

Film exit

1. _____ 2. _____ 3. _____ Drying element

16. What is the purpose of including a lead collimator inside the dental tubehead?
   a. To direct the x-ray beam
   b. To restrict the size and shape of the x-ray beam
   c. To remove the low energy x-rays from the beam
   d. To protect the reproductive tissues from scatter radiation

17. What is the term to describe the point in radiation exposure when cell death occurs?
   a. Latent period
   b. Period of injury
   c. Recovery period
   d. Cumulative exposures

18. Which radiology item is replaced by a digital sensor?
   a. X-ray beam
   b. Film processor
   c. Intraoral dental film
   d. X-ray machine

19. When exposing intraoral radiographs, in which the patient's right is on your left, the identification dot on the film will be positioned where?
   a. Facing out and toward the incisal/occlusal
   b. Facing out away from the incisal/occlusal
   c. Facing in and toward the incisal/occlusal
   d. Facing in and away from the incisal/occlusal

20. In which two lengths are PIDs typically available?
   a. 6 and 12 inches
   b. 12 and 24 inches
   c. 8 and 16 inches
   d. 12 and 16 inches

21. How should the film be placed when exposing a mandibular occlusal radiograph?
    a. White side facing the lingual of the teeth
    b. White side up between the occlusal surfaces of the maxillary and mandibular teeth
    c. Colored side facing the lingual of the teeth
    d. Colored side up between the occlusal surfaces of the maxillary and mandibular teeth

22. Direct digital imaging involves digitizing an existing x-ray film using a CCD camera. Indirect digital imaging is superior to direct digital imaging.
    a. Both statements are correct.
    b. Both statements are false.
    c. Statement 1 is correct; statement 2 is incorrect.
    d. Statement 1 is incorrect; statement 2 is correct.

23. Which of the following refers to operator protection during radiographic procedures?
    a. Avoid the primary beam.
    b. Use a lead apron.
    c. Determine the need for radiographs.
    d. Avoid retakes.

24. Which landmark would be found in the mandibular molar exposure?
    a. Inverted Y
    b. Mylohyoid ridge
    c. Mental foramen
    d. External oblique ridge

25. Which form of radiation is found in the environment and includes cosmic and terrestrial radiation?
    a. Characteristic
    b. Scatter
    c. Braking
    d. Background

26. Which of the following statements is TRUE as it relates to the direct theory of radiation?
    a. Cell damage results when ionizing radiation directly hits critical areas or targets within the cell.
    b. Direct injuries from exposure to ionizing radiation occur frequently but seldom do noticeable damage.
    c. Most x-ray photons are absorbed by the cell and cause little or no damage.
    d. Indirect injuries occur at the same rate as direct injuries from exposure to ionizing radiation.

27. Which cells are affected when radiation exposure produces mutations to future generations?
    a. Biologic
    b. Somatic
    c. Genetic
    d. Cumulative

28. Which body tissue listed is the most sensitive to radiation exposure?
    a. Small blood vessels
    b. Bone marrow
    c. Thyroid gland
    d. Lymph glands

29. When converting to digital radiography, which aspect of the process remains a concern for dental offices?
    a. Use of a lead apron
    b. Chemical disposal
    c. Trash disposal
    d. Missing exposures

30. Which exposure method would produce the smallest patient dose of radiation?
   a. E-speed film
   b. F-speed film
   c. G-speed film
   d. Digital sensor

31. A bite-wing image shows the _____ of both the _____ and _____.
   a. entire tooth, maxilla, mandible
   b. crowns, right, left
   c. crowns, maxilla, mandible
   d. entire tooth, posterior, anterior

32. The collimator:
   a. is always round.
   b. restricts the size and shape of the x-ray beam.
   c. is a solid piece of aluminum.
   d. is fitted within the copper stem beneath the molybdenum cup.

33. After a lead apron is used, it should be:
   a. disinfected.
   b. folded and stored.
   c. hung up or laid on a rounded bar.
   d. both A and C.

34. The_____ image provides a wide view of the maxilla and mandible.
   a. bite-wing
   b. periapical
   c. panoramic
   d. cephalometric

35. _____ film can be used in cassettes.
   a. Intensifying
   b. Panoramic
   c. Extraoral
   d. Intraoral

36. To increase the contrast on a radiograph, one should _____ the kilovoltage peak.
   a. Decrease
   b. Increase

37. A tissue that lies within the primary dental beam and is very radio-sensitive is the _____.
   a. Tongue
   b. Cornea
   c. Thyroid
   d. Inner ear

38. A _____ radiograph provides a view that shows the tooth crown, root tip, and surrounding structures of a specific area.
   a. bite-wing
   b. periapical
   c. panoramic
   d. cephalometric

39. In a dental practice in which many HIV-positive patients are treated, the film rollers in the automatic processor should be _____.
   a. scrubbed with an abrasive cleaner every day
   b. autoclaved every day
   c. disinfected after every use
   d. treated in the usual accepted manner

40. _____ is an example of a patient protection technique used before x-ray exposure.
   a. Proper image processing
   b. Proper prescribing of radiographs
   c. A lead apron
   d. A thyroid collar

41. Inherent filtration in the dental x-ray tubehead: _____.
   a. includes filtration that takes place when the primary beam passes through the glass window of the x-ray tube, the insulating oil, and the tubehead seal
   b. includes the placement of aluminum discs in the path of the x-ray beam between the collimator and the tubehead seal
   c. alone meets the standards regulated by state and federal law
   d. is equivalent to approximately 5.0 mm of aluminum

42. Before radiation exposure for a minor, informed consent _____.
   a. must be obtained from an adult
   b. must be obtained from a legal guardian
   c. must be obtained from the patient
   d. may be waived if the patient has insurance

43. Rules of radiation protection for the operator include all of the following EXCEPT _____.
   a. never stand in the direct line of the primary beam
   b. always stand behind a lead barrier or a proper thickness of drywall
   c. never stand closer than 3 feet from the x-ray unit during an exposure
   d. monitor radiation exposure

44. Personnel monitoring of radiation exposure _____.
   a. identifies the location of exposure to primary beams
   b. identifies occupational exposure to radiation
   c. measures the amount of exposure for each patient
   d. alerts the operator when the maximum amount of exposure for the month has been reached

45. The acronym for the permitted lifetime accumulated dose is _____.
   a. MPD, maximum permissible dose
   b. MPD, maximum possible dose
   c. MAD, maximum accumulated dose
   d. MAD, maximum allowable dose

46. To prevent occupational exposure to radiation, which is the most critical for a dental radiographer?
   a. Maintain an adequate distance.
   b. Have proper positioning of the patient.
   c. Use proper shielding.
   d. Avoid exposure to the primary beam.

47. All of the following relate to operator safety EXCEPT _____.
    a. leakage from the tubehead
    b. distance from the source
    c. concrete walls
    d. paralleling technique

48. From which of the following metals is the filter made?
    a. Lead
    b. Copper
    c. Tungsten
    d. Aluminum

49. Thermionic emission occurs at the filament on the cathode and is controlled by the:
    a. mA setting.
    b. kVp setting.
    c. focal spot.
    d. exposure button.

50. An increase in exposure time will result in a radiograph that is:
    a. more dense.
    b. lighter.
    c. low contrast.
    d. short scale.

51. Which of the following prevents further penetration of the primary beam?
    a. Film packet
    b. Film cassette
    c. Lead foil
    d. Intensifying screen

52. Which of the following is a true statement regarding radiation and patient protection?
    a. X-rays are routinely prescribed for 6-month recall patients.
    b. Round collimators are preferred over rectangular collimators.
    c. A patient may hold the film in place when XCPs are not available.
    d. The benefit of dental x-rays outweighs the risk of ionizing radiation.

53. Which of the following methods is LEAST effective in helping a patient understand the value of dental radiographs?
    a. An oral presentation
    b. Printed literature
    c. Allowing the patient to observe radiographs being taken
    d. A discussion with the dentist

54. Who determines the number, type, and frequency of dental radiographs?
    a. Dental hygienist
    b. Dental assistant
    c. Dentist
    d. American Dental Association

55. When a patient who refuses to have dental radiographs taken offers to sign a waiver of responsibility, what is the most appropriate action?
    a. Inform the patient that the dental staff cannot consent to negligent care.
    b. Make a note in the chart that the patient has refused x-rays.
    c. Tell the dentist that the patient will have them next time.
    d. Ask the patient to get radiographs from his/her previous dentist.

56. Areas in the oral cavity most likely to cause a gag reflex when stimulated include the _____.
    a. soft palate and lateral borders of the tongue
    b. floor of the mouth and posterior of the tongue
    c. hard palate and base of the tongue
    d. posterior one-third of the tongue and palatoglossal arch

57. Proper film size for an edentulous patient is_____.
    a. No. 0
    b. No. 1
    c. No. 2
    d. No. 3

58. Which of the following describes one reason for the difficulty encountered in trying to expose an image of a tooth undergoing an endodontic procedure?
    a. Patient movement
    b. Excessive salivation
    c. Equipment used in the endodontic procedure
    d. Poor visualization of the canals

59. Proper handling of replenisher solution includes: _____.
    a. replenishing both developer and fixer
    b. waiting for oxidation to occur prior to replenishing the tanks
    c. replenishing 6 ounces of fixer solution daily
    d. replenishing 3 ounces of developer daily

60. Which of the following are ideal temperature and humidity levels for film storage?
    a. 50-70 degrees F; 30% to 50%
    b. 60-80 degrees F; 50% to 60%
    c. 70-90 degrees F; 60% to 70%
    d. below 50 degrees F; 0% to 30%

61. The hardening agent in fixer solution is _____.
    a. acetic acid
    b. potassium alum
    c. sodium sulfite
    d. thiosulfate

62. The GBX-2 safelight filter by Kodak is considered appropriate to develop which of the following types of films?
    a. Intraoral
    b. Extraoral
    c. Both intra and extraoral

63. Thermometers for manual processing should be placed in the _____.
   a. developer solution
   b. water bath
   c. fixer solution
   d. either a or c

64. Residual gelatin and dirt can be removed from the rollers of the automatic processor with which of the following?
   a. A cleaning film
   b. A soft cloth, soap, and cold water
   c. A solution of ammonia and water
   d. A solution of sodium hypochlorite and water

65. Which of the following does not affect the life of processing solutions?
   a. The number of films being processed
   b. Care in solution preparation
   c. Type of safelight filter used
   d. Age of the solutions

66. Automatic film processing has the following advantage over manual film processing EXCEPT which of the following?
   a. It saves time.
   b. Radiographs are of higher quality.
   c. Several patients' films can be processed at the same time.
   d. It requires less maintenance.

67. The purpose of the stirring rod in a manual processing tank is to _____.
   a. agitate the water bath only
   b. agitate the fixer only
   c. agitate the developer only
   d. agitate the chemicals and equalize the temperature of the solution

68. A film duplicator is a _____.
   a. source of x-radiation
   b. light source
   c. form of safe light
   d. print process

69. When placing duplicating film over the arranged radiographs, in which direction is the emulsion is placed?
   a. Up
   b. Down
   c. It does not matter

70. Unused developer solution may be considered hazardous because _____.
   a. it is an inhalation hazard
   b. it is a skin irritant
   c. it has a relatively low pH
   d. it has a high pH

71. Silver recovered from used fixer and rinse water solutions must be disposed of by which of the following means?
    a. In the sanitary sewer
    b. In the septic tank
    c. Picked up and disposed of via an appropriate waste management service
    d. In a biohazard bag

72. Designing and seeing to it that a hazard communication plan is in place and properly adhered to is the responsibility of _____.
    a. the dental assistant
    b. the dental staff
    c. the hazard communication officer
    d. the employer

73. The term MSDS (material safety data sheets) is being replaced by which of the following terms?
    a. DS
    b. MDS
    c. MSHA
    d. SDS

74. Which type of material can cause irritating skin, eyes, or lungs and can cause illness or death?
    a. Toxic
    b. Infectious
    c. Hazardous
    d. Harmful

75. The Hazardous Communication Standard is sometimes also called the _____.
    a. Employer Standard for Staff Protection
    b. Employee Right to Know Standard
    c. Employee Protocol Manual
    d. Employee Protection Plan

76. According to GHS, all chemicals will contain the following information EXCEPT which of the following?
    a. Signal word
    b. Pictogram
    c. Hazard statement
    d. Date of manufacture

77. Repair of dental radiography equipment is done by which of the following?
    a. A qualified technician
    b. The dental assistant
    c. The dentist
    d. All staff

78. Following processing, fresh and properly stored film will appear _____.
    a. clear with a slight blue tint
    b. cloudy with a blue tint
    c. fogged
    d. totally black

79. Testing the safelight should be done at which frequency?
a. Annually
b. Twice annually
c. Monthly
d. Depends on the volume of radiography being done

80. EPA-registered chemical germicides labeled as *sterilants* are classified as
_____.
a. high-level disinfectants
b. intermediate-level disinfectants
c. low-level disinfectants

81. Following an exposure, beam alignment devices are placed for processing by _____ hands.
a. gloved
b. ungloved

82. Which describes the level of disinfectant appropriate for disinfection of a sensor?
a. High-level disinfectant
b. Intermediate-level disinfectant
c. Low-level disinfectant

83. Where in the dental practice would a list of all the chemicals used in the processing of dental films be found?
a. In the employee handbook
b. In the engineering controls document
c. In the written Hazard Communication Plan
d. In the OSHA Bloodborne Pathogen Standard

84. Safety data sheets have _____ sections.
a. 4
b. 5
c. 9
d. 16

85. Which is the method used to prevent cross-contamination during use of a digital sensor?
a. Heat sterilization
b. Disinfection
c. Barrier technique
d. Cold sterilization
e. B and C

86. Infection control practiced during exposure involves all of the following EXCEPT _____.
a. disposal of contaminated items
b. drying of the exposed receptor
c. reassembling of the beam alignment device
d. A, B, and C

87. Washing with an alcohol-based product until hands are dry describes which term?
a. Standard handwashing
b. Antiseptic hand rub
c. Routine handwashing
d. Disinfecting hand rub

88. An instrument that contacts mucous membranes but does not penetrate soft tissue or bone is considered_____.
    a. critical
    b. semicritical
    c. noncritical
    d. semicritical and noncritical

89. Which procedure must be performed before gloving?
    a. Preparing the beam alignment devices
    b. Adjusting the headrest
    c. Placing the lead apron
    d. B and C

90. Which choice describes recommended protocol for asking a parent to assist with an uncooperative child?
    a. Asking the parent to hold the child in his/her lap and covering the child with a lead apron
    b. Asking the parent to hold the child in his/her lap and covering the parent with a lead apron
    c. Asking the parent to hold the child in his/her lap and individually covering both with a lead apron.

91. Which choice describes a single-use item in a radiographic procedure?
    a. Film mount
    b. Cotton rolls
    c. Beam alignment devices
    d. Patient chart

92. Examples of items to clean, disinfect, and/or protect with surface barriers in dental radiography are:_____.
    a. the tube head
    b. the exposure panel
    c. a beam alignment device
    d. A, B, and C
    e. A and B

93. Which is the first step in handling film with barrier envelopes during processing?
    a. Put on gloves.
    b. Tear open the barrier envelope.
    c. Place the container with contaminated films next to the towel.
    d. Place a disposable towel on the work surface.

94. In a dental radiographic procedure, which is the LEAST likely mode of disease transmission?
    a. Bloodborne
    b. Airborne
    c. Indirect
    d. Sexual

95. The greatest infection control risk of the dental professional in radiographic procedures is from _____.
    a. exposing the dental films
    b. handing exposed dental films
    c. the fixing process
    d. mounting the radiographs

96. When dental films not in barrier sleeves are exposed and removed from the oral cavity, they are
_____.
    a. dropped into the disposable container and transported for processing
    b. placed on the counter until all films are exposed
    c. wiped off prior to being placed in the disposable container
    d. placed in the right lab coat pocket

97. Film holders should be _____.
    a. heat-tolerant
    b. disposable
    c. disinfected
    d. placed in a sterilization pouch and kept in the patient's record for reuse after sterilization
    e. A or B

98. Which describes appropriate protocol for single-use devices in a radiography procedure?
    a. Disinfecting prior to reusing
    b. Discarding the item
    c. Sterilizing before reusing
    d. Giving to the patient
    e. A and C

99. How must the counter and or work area be prepared before the patient is seated?
    a. Disinfected
    b. Barriers placed
    c. Washed with a high-level disinfectant only
    d. None of the above
    e. A and B

100. In this panoramic radiograph, which of the following statements is TRUE?
    a. The permanent mandibular second molars are erupted.
    b. There is no evidence of mandibular third molars.
    c. There are malpositioned maxillary canines.
    d. The primary maxillary first molars are still present.

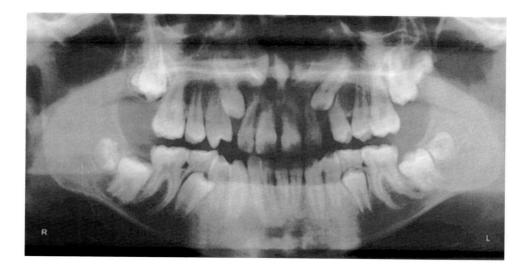

Infection Control

Directions: Select the response that best answers each of the following questions. Only one response is correct.

1. If you opt not to receive a hepatitis B vaccination, you will be required to sign:
   a. a waiver that you will not ever request the vaccine
   b. a waiver that if you change your mind you will assume the cost of the vaccine
   c. an informed refusal that is kept on file in the dental office
   d. an informed refusal that is sent to OSHA

2. All dental professionals must use surgical masks and protective eyewear to protect the eyes and face:
   a. only during surgical procedures
   b. only when treating patients of potential risk
   c. whenever spatter and aerosolized sprays of blood and saliva are likely
   d. as an option

3. All dental assistants involved in the direct provision of patient care must undergo routine training in:
   a. infection control, safety issues, and hazard communication
   b. charting, taking patients' vital signs, and using the office intercom system
   c. infection control, uniform sizing, and ordering of disposables
   d. hazardous waste management, charting, and application of dental dam

4. _____ occurs from a person previously contracting a disease and then recovering.
   a. Naturally acquired immunity
   b. Active natural immunity
   c. Artificially acquired immunity
   d. Inherited immunity

5. _____ immunity occurs when a vaccination is administered and the body forms antibodies in response to the vaccine.
   a. Active natural
   b. Active artificial
   c. Passive natural
   d. Passive artificial

6. A latent infection is best exemplified by which of the following?
   a. hepatitis A
   b. cold sore
   c. common cold
   d. pneumonia

7. Which of the following exemplifies an acute infection?
   a. hepatitis C
   b. cold sore
   c. common cold
   d. hepatitis B

8. Microorganisms that produce disease in humans are known as:
   a. nonpathogenic
   b. pathogens
   c. pasteurized
   d. aerobes

9. When should an alcohol hand rub be used for routine dentistry?
   a. anytime
   b. immediately after handwashing
   c. in the absence of visible soil
   d. immediately before handwashing

10. An infection that occurs when the body's ability to resist diseases is weakened is:
   a. a chronic infection
   b. a latent infection
   c. an acute infection
   d. an opportunistic infection

11. A disposable air/water syringe tip is to be:
   a. used on no more than three patients before being replaced
   b. cleaned, sterilized, and reused
   c. cleaned, disinfected, and reused
   d. used on one patient and then discarded

12. The transmission of a disease through the skin, as with cuts or punctures, is _____ transmission.
   a. airborne
   b. parenteral
   c. indirect
   d. spatter

13. Which of the following would be considered the best method for determining whether there is proper sterilization function by a sterilizer?
   a. chemically treated tape used on packages that changes color
   b. viewing the temperature gauge
   c. biological spore test through a monitoring system
   d. measuring the pressure

14. When leaving a patient at chairside to retrieve a supply item, which barrier should be removed and replaced after returning to the patient?
   a. mask
   b. eyewear
   c. gloves
   d. protective clothing

15. Protective eyewear should have:
   a. extra-thick lenses
   b. tinted lenses
   c. solid side shields
   d. spring-loaded ear rests

16. What is the most serious reaction to gloves?
   a. allergic contact dermatitis
   b. irritant contact dermatitis
   c. anaphylaxis
   d. candidiasis

17. Which of the following is regulated medical waste?
   a. used examination gloves
   b. used patient bib
   c. a used anesthetic needle
   d. x-ray wrappers

18. The microbes that contaminate the hands after touching surfaces are referred to as:
   a. transient flora
   b. resistant flora
   c. anaerobic flora
   d. resident flora

19. During which of the following procedures would you use sterile surgical gloves?
   a. placement of a composite
   b. removal of a suture
   c. all bonding procedures
   d. mandibular resection

20. Which of the following statements is an inappropriate action for postexposure medical evaluation and follow-up?
   a. The employer must send the employee for medical evaluation, for which the employee must assume the cost.
   b. Give a copy of the OSHA standard to the health care professional.
   c. File an incident report.
   d. Assure that test results of the source individual are given to the health care professional and that the health care professional informs the employee of these results confidentially.

21. Which of the following is a cause of sterilization failure?
   a. adequate space between packages in the autoclave
   b. using paper bags in a steam sterilizer
   c. using closed containers in steam or chemical vapor sterilizer
   d. using distilled water in a steam sterilizer

22. To prevent contamination of surfaces, which of the following techniques should be used?
   a. Place utility gloves before placement of appropriate surface covers.
   b. Apply appropriate surface covers before the surfaces have a chance to become contaminated with patient material.
   c. Place each cover surface directly under the cassette so the entire surface is not cluttered with protective covers.
   d. Always clean the underlying protected surface with a disinfectant.

23. An emergency action plan may be communicated orally if the workplace has fewer than _____ employees.
   a. 3
   b. 5
   c. 7
   d. 10

24. What is the maximum volume that a single container of alcohol-based hand rub solution placed within a dental treatment room can legally have?
   a. 250 mL
   b. 400 mL
   c. 2.0 L
   d. 5.0 L

25. Which of the following surfaces need *not* be cleaned and disinfected before each patient appointment?
   a. drawer pulls and top edges of drawers that may be used
   b. floors
   c. high-volume evacuation connector
   d. handpiece connectors

26. Which of the following is *least* important in protecting dental instruments?
   a. clean as soon as possible after use
   b. rinse well after cleaning
   c. use distilled or deionized water in steam sterilizers
   d. dry items before processing through steam under pressure sterilizers

27. Which of the following microbes on the hands are the most important in the spread of diseases?
   a. transient flora
   b. resistant flora
   c. anaerobic flora
   d. resident flora

28. When alcohol hand rubs are used all day long why is it important to wash the hands every so often?
   a. because alcohol hand rubs do not kill the microbes as well as does handwashing
   b. to remove the buildup of glove material, sweat, and dead microbes
   c. the residual handwashing agent left on the hands makes it easier to put on gloves
   d. most alcohol hand rubs slowly damage latex gloves

29. When should protective clothing be changed during the day?
   a. when it is visibly soiled
   b. for every patient
   c. after using the high-speed handpiece
   d. after treating patients older than age 65 years

30. When an assistant transfers a microbe from one patient to his or her hand and then to another patient's mouth, this transmission is referred to as:
   a. direct contact
   b. indirect contact
   c. airborne transmission
   d. droplet transmission

31. _____ is a protein manufactured in the body that binds to and destroys microbes and other antigens.
   a. An antibiotic
   b. An antibody
   c. A microbe
   d. An allergen

32. When should the surgical face mask be changed?
    a. after every other patient
    b. only if it becomes wet
    c. for every patient
    d. only after treating patients older than age 65 years

33. What particles are involved in airborne transmission?
    a. aerosols
    b. spatter
    c. droplets
    d. splashes

34. Why should instruments be packaged before placing in a sterilizer?
    a. to prevent rusting of the instruments
    b. to protect the instruments from becoming recontaminated during storage
    c. to keep the white residue from "water spots" off the instruments
    d. to eliminate any sparks if the instruments should touch the inside of the sterilizer chamber

35. Recommendations concerning gloves would fall under which of the following categories of infection control practices that directly relate to dental radiography procedures?
    a. Surface disinfection
    b. Protective attire and barrier techniques
    c. Sterilization or disinfection of instruments
    d. Maintenance of the environment

36. Protective clothing:
    a. must protect skin, work clothes, and undergarments
    b. must be taken home every day and laundered
    c. must be worn to and from work
    d. must be disposable

37. Amalgam contains which of the following hazardous materials?
    a. glutaraldehyde
    b. acetic acid
    c. mercury
    d. acetone

38. Special protective eyewear is to be worn when:
    a. using a curing light
    b. taking x-rays
    c. mixing amalgam
    d. placing a capped anesthetic needle into a sharps container

39. A latex allergy is caused by sensitivity to:
    a. cornstarch (glove powder)
    b. excessive amounts of one's sweat that builds up beneath the gloves
    c. proteins present in the latex obtained from the rubber tree
    d. the cardboard material in the boxes that contain the latex gloves

40. Which of the following best explains the relationship between latex allergies and glove powder (cornstarch)?
   a. The glove powder protects the wearer from all allergic reactions.
   b. The latex allergy is actually caused by the cornstarch itself rather than the latex in gloves.
   c. There is no relationship.
   d. The powder can spread latex allergens when it becomes airborne.

41. When using medical latex or vinyl gloves:
   a. gloves may be rewashed between patients and reused until damaged.
   b. nonsterile gloves are recommended for examinations and nonsurgical procedures.
   c. hands should not be washed before gloving.
   d. hands should not be washed between patients.

42. _____ is defined as the absence of pathogens, or disease-causing microorganisms.
   a. Antiseptic
   b. Antibiotic
   c. Antiinfective
   d. Asepsis

43. Antiseptic refers to:
   a. the absence of pathogens, or disease-causing microorganisms
   b. a substance that inhibits the growth of bacteria
   c. a chemical used to disinfect operatory surfaces
   d. the act of sterilizing

44. According to OSHA's Hazard Communication Standard, the list of hazardous chemicals in the office needs to be cross-referenced to the:
   a. patients' appointment schedules for each day
   b. Safety Data Sheets
   c. schedule for disinfecting operatory surfaces
   d. Exposure Control Plan

45. Which of the following agents is *not* tuberculocidal?
   a. iodophor
   b. quaternary ammonium compound
   c. phenolic
   d. glutaraldehyde

46. When can a liquid sterilant/high-level disinfectant achieve sterilization?
   a. only when the solution is used at temperatures above 121°C
   b. when the solution is used only for longer exposure times
   c. as soon as the minimal exposure time is reached
   d. only when the solution is used under pressure

47. Which of the following may be used for surface disinfectant disinfection in the dental office?
   a. iodophors
   b. ethyl alcohol
   c. isopropyl alcohol
   d. iodine

48. Autoclaves are preset to reach a maximum steam temperature of ____ degrees Fahrenheit.
   a. 500
   b. 350
   c. 250
   d. 400

49. The best way to avoid contracting a bloodborne disease in the office is to:
   a. not shake hands with patients
   b. wear a mask with all patients
   c. handle sharps carefully
   d. use a preprocedure mouthrinse on all patients

50. Which of the following is considered to be a semicritical instrument in radiography?
   a. the exposure button
   b. the x-ray control panel
   c. the lead apron
   d. the x-ray film–holding device

51. Which of the following is a work practice control as described by OSHA?
   a. using a sharps container
   b. using a one-handed scoop technique to recap an anesthetic needle
   c. using a rubber dam
   d. using a high–volume evacuator

52. Which method of sterilization requires good room ventilation?
   a. steam under pressure
   b. cold chemical/immersion disinfection
   c. unsaturated chemical vapor
   d. flash sterilization

53. OSHA requires which of the following documents to be present in every dental facility?
   a. the names, addresses, and professions of all the patients seen every day
   b. the monthly total amounts paid to dental laboratories
   c. an exposure control plan
   d. the treatment plans and outcomes of treatment for all patients older than age 65 years

54. Which government agency requires employers to protect their employees from exposure to blood and saliva at work?
   a. FDA
   b. EPA
   c. CDC
   d. OSHA

55. Improper cleaning or sterilizing of reusable hand instruments can contribute to which pathway of cross-contamination in the office?
   a. patient to dental team
   b. patient to patient
   c. dental team to patient
   d. community to office

56. The main publication for all OSHA information is the:
   a. *Federal Register*
   b. *Journal of the American Dental Association*
   c. *Morbidity and Mortality Weekly Report*
   d. *Dental Products Report*

57. From the list below, select the best procedure for caring for orthodontic wire.
   a. steam under pressure with emulsion
   b. steam under pressure without emulsion
   c. sharps container
   d. spray/wipe/spray with surface disinfectant

58. From the list below, select the best procedure for caring for a pair of crown and collar scissors.
   a. steam under pressure with emulsion
   b. steam under pressure without emulsion
   c. cold chemical/immersion
   d. spray/wipe/spray with surface disinfectant

59. From the list below, select the best procedure for caring for a pair of surgical suction tips.
   a. steam under pressure with emulsion
   b. steam under pressure without emulsion
   c. cold chemical/immersion
   d. spray/wipe/spray with surface disinfectant

60. Which of the following is the recommended scheme for immunization against hepatitis B?
   a. injections at 0, 1, and 6 months
   b. an injection now and then another one in 1 month
   c. injections at 0, 1, and 3 months
   d. an injection now and another one 6 months later

61. From the list below, select the best procedure for caring for a mandrel.
   a. steam under pressure with emulsion
   b. steam under pressure without emulsion
   c. cold chemical/immersion
   d. discard

62. The intent of handwashing is to remove:
   a. transient flora and soil
   b. normal flora and soil
   c. transient and normal flora
   d. soil

63. From the list below, select the best procedure for caring for a pair of protective glasses.
   a. steam under pressure with emulsion
   b. steam under pressure without emulsion
   c. chemical disinfection
   d. dry heat sterilization

64. What is the active agent in hand rubs acceptable for use in dental offices?
   a. triclosan
   b. chlorhexidine
   c. iodophor
   d. alcohol

65. Which type of sterilization used in the dental office requires the longest processing time?
    a. steam autoclave
    b. chemical vapor
    c. dry heat sterilization
    d. chemical liquid sterilization

66. What is required by the postexposure evaluation section of the Bloodborne Pathogens Standard?
    a. All patients exposed to an HIV-positive or hepatitis B–positive dental office employee must be evaluated for their bloodborne disease status.
    b. Employees exposed to a patient's blood or saliva must be evaluated for their bloodborne disease status.
    c. An OSHA inspector must evaluate employers and employees exposed to a patient's blood or saliva for their bloodborne disease status.
    d. All employees must be vaccinated against hepatitis B to prevent disease after an exposure.

67. Instruments have been in a liquid sterilant for 2 hours. The assistant adds another batch of instruments. Which of the following statements addresses this situation?
    a. Two completion times will be used: one for the first set of instrument and the other for the second batch.
    b. The total time will be 24 hours for the entire batch.
    c. The total time will be 1 hour for the entire batch.
    d. Retiming must begin again once the second batch has been added to the original instruments.

68. According to the Bloodborne Pathogens Standard, who must provide gloves, masks, eyeglasses, and protective clothing to the dental assistant in the office?
    a. The dental assistant must supply his or her own protective equipment.
    b. The employing dentist must supply this protective equipment.
    c. OSHA must supply this protective equipment.
    d. The dental assistant must provide protective clothing, and the employer dentist must provide gloves, masks, and protective eyewear.

69. Which of the following methods of precleaning dental instruments should be avoided?
    a. instrument washing machines
    b. rinsing in a holding solution
    c. hand scrubbing
    d. ultrasonic cleaning

70. One of the main the purposes of the Hazard Communication Standard is to require:
    a. that employees are able to communicate their concerns about disease exposure in the office
    b. patients to inform health care workers if they are HIV positive
    c. that the hazards of chemicals are evaluated and that information concerning their hazards is transmitted to employers and employees
    d. employers to protect employees from being contaminated with patients' body fluids during all work activities

71. Which of the following organizations make laws that are associated with fines for noncompliance?
    a. OSAP
    b. OSHA
    c. CDC
    d. ADA

72. The last item(s) of the PPEs to be put on before patient treatment begins:
   a. is the gown
   b. is the mask
   c. are gloves
   d. are eyeglasses

73. Heavy utility gloves should be used:
   a. for all intraoral procedures
   b. for radiographic processing
   c. for entering data on the computer
   d. to work with contaminated instruments

74. Which of the following types of germicides can be used as a high-level disinfectant or a sterilant by following the manufacturer's guidelines for immersion time?
   a. iodophors
   b. glutaraldehyde
   c. phenolic
   d. triclosan

75. The 2012 update of the OSHA Hazard Communication Standard changed the name of Material Safety Data Sheets to:
   a. Exposure Determination Sheets
   b. Safety Data Sheets
   c. Chemical Information Sheets
   d. Hazard Caution Sheets

76. The process that kills disease-causing microorganisms, but not necessarily all microbial life, is defined as:
   a. precleaning
   b. sterilization
   c. disinfection
   d. cleaning

77. The best way to determine that sterilization has actually occurred is to use:
   a. process integrators
   b. biologic monitors
   c. process indicators
   d. color-changing sterilization bags or tape

78. The rule that requires employers to do certain things to prevent employees from being exposed to human body fluids at work is called the:
   a. Universal Precautions Standard
   b. Hazard Communications Standard
   c. Medical Device Standard
   d. Bloodborne Pathogens Standard

79. Patient care instruments are categorized into various classifications. Into which classification would instruments such as impression trays, dental mouth mirror, and amalgam condenser be placed?
   a. critical
   b. semicritical
   c. noncritical

80. Which of the following is *least* effective in minimizing the amount of dental aerosols and spatter generated during treatment?
    a. preprocedural mouth rinse
    b. saliva ejectors
    c. rubber dams
    d. high-volume evacuation

81. Which of the following microbes will remain alive after exposure to an intermediate-level disinfectant?
    a. bacterial spores
    b. tuberculosis agent
    c. all viruses
    d. all fungi

82. Which of the following is the *least* appropriate PPE for cleaning and disinfecting a dental treatment room?
    a. mask
    b. utility gloves
    c. latex examination gloves
    d. protective eyewear

83. The OSHA Bloodborne Pathogens Standard is designed to prevent which of the following diseases?
    a. strep throat
    b. influenza
    c. hepatitis C
    d. oral candidiasis (thrush)

84. OSHA indicates that one way to prevent exposure to human body fluids is to use engineering controls. What is an engineering control?
    a. Altering the manner in which a task is performed
    b. Maintaining building air conditioning and heating systems in good working order
    c. Hiring a licensed engineer to review the mechanical aspects of the building
    d. Using a device to isolate or remove a hazard

85. The Organization for Safety, Asepsis and Prevention identifies the classification of clinical touch surfaces to include which of the following?
    a. sinks, handpiece holders, and countertops
    b. light handles, dental unit controls, and chair switches
    c. unit master switch, fixed cabinetry, and patient record
    d. telephone, assistant stool, and fixed cabinetry

86. Chemicals that destroy or inactivate most species of pathogenic microorganisms on inanimate surfaces are called:
    a. disinfectants
    b. sterilants
    c. antiseptics
    d. antibiotics

87. According to the OSHA Hazard Communication Standard, who determines the hazards of a chemical?
    a. employer
    b. employees
    c. manufacturer
    d. distributor

88. When a denture is to be repaired by a commercial laboratory, it should be:
   a. disinfected before being sent out
   b. packaged and sent to the laboratory for later disinfection
   c. disinfected after being received back from the laboratory
   d. disinfected before being sent out and after being received back from the laboratory

89. A victim who feels the effects of a chemical spill immediately, with symptoms of dizziness, headache, nausea, and vomiting, is experiencing:
   a. chronic chemical toxicity
   b. acute chemical toxicity
   c. chemical resistance
   d. mild exposure

90. _____ is considered regulated waste and requires special disposal.
   a. Human tissue
   b. Food
   c. Gauze damp with saliva
   d. Used patient bib

91. The office safety supervisor should check the contents of the emergency kit to determine that the contents are in place and within the expiration date:
   a. weekly
   b. monthly
   c. biannually
   d. annually

92. Which of the following is to be used for cleaning and disinfecting blood-contaminated operatory surfaces?
   a. an intermediate-level disinfectant
   b. a low-level disinfectant
   c. a liquid sterilant
   d. an antiseptic

93. All waste containers that hold potentially infectious materials must be:
   a. made of see-through material
   b. labeled with the biohazard symbol
   c. colored yellow
   d. labeled as infectious waste

94. The OSHA Hazard Communications Standard requires employers to do all *except:*
   a. tell employees about the identity and hazards of chemicals in the workplace
   b. implement a hazard communication program
   c. maintain accurate and thorough SDS records
   d. submit annual hair sample results of all employees

95. A dental health care worker transfers a small amount of cavity medication into a smaller container for use on a patient at chairside. A new label must be placed on that container if:
   a. more material is required during the course of treating that patient
   b. the chemical material is not used up at the conclusion of an 8-hour work shift
   c. the patient recently tested positive for HIV
   d. no SDS can be found on file for that material

96. The microbial accumulation on the inside walls of dental unit waterlines is best referred to as:
    a. a culture
    b. a biofilm
    c. a probiotic
    d. an antibiotic

97. The ADA, OSAP, and CDC recommend that the dental assistant:
    a. flush the dental unit waterlines for 30 seconds each morning and again at the end of the day
    b. flush the dental unit waterlines for 20 to 30 seconds each morning and between patients
    c. flush the dental unit waterlines 60 seconds each morning and 30 seconds after treating an HIV-infected patient
    d. flush the dental unit waterlines for 30 seconds each hour of the day

98. For instruments to be sterilized, they must first be:
    a. placed in sterilization pouches
    b. cleaned of blood and debris
    c. inspected for rust or corrosion
    d. treated with surgical milk

99. Who is required by the Occupational Safety and Health Administration to pay for the protective clothing used by dental assistants?
    a. the dental assistants
    b. the employer
    c. the patients (It is figured into their bill.)
    d. the manufacturer of the clothing

100. According to the Occupational Safety and Health Administration (OSHA), who pays for the OSHA-required training for employees in the dental office?
    a. the employer
    b. the employees
    c. the patients (It is figured into their bill.)
    d. the school from which the employees graduated

Answer Keys and Rationales

TEST 3

General Chairside

1. A patient displaying hypertension would have a blood pressure of about:
   d. Hypertension is considered to be a blood pressure of 140/90 mm Hg and above. Normal blood pressure for an adult is less than 120/80 mm Hg. Blood pressure of 100/70 mm Hg is considered low blood pressure and dangerous. Blood pressure of 110/90 mm Hg is also considered low but not so low to cause alarm.
   CAT: Collection and Recording of Clinical Data

2. A patient presents appearing "flushed" and states that he has an infection. Which temperature would most likely be measured?
   d. If a patient presented with the symptoms as listed, the temperature would likely be higher than 99.6° F; thus, the best answer is 102°F. A normal temperature is 98.6°F. A temperature of 93°F is low considering the normal temperature and would not indicate that an infection is present.
   CAT: Collection & Recording of Clinical Data

3. The normal blood pressure classification for adults is:
   a. A normal blood pressure for an adult is less than 120/80 mm Hg. High blood pressure is rated over the norm based on the individual patient such as 130/70 mm Hg. Blood pressures reaching 145/90 and 155/115 mm Hg may indicate hypertension.
   CAT: Collection and Recording of Clinical Data

4. The most common site for taking a patient's pulse when performing cardiopulmonary resuscitation is the:
   b. The carotid artery is the most common site for taking a patient's pulse when administering CPR. This pulse is found by placing two fingers alongside the patient's larynx on the side of the neck nearest you.

The radial artery is in the inner wrist area and used to take the pulse before dental procedures. The brachial artery is on the inner fold of the arm used for blood pressure. The femoral artery is in the inner thing of the leg and not typically used in a dental office.
CAT: Prevention and Management of Emergencies

5. Consent is:
   d. Consent is a voluntary acceptance or agreement to what is planned or done by another person. Consent is given freely by the patient. Consent to treat is for all applicable procedures, not just related to surgical procedures. Consent is used on all patients regardless of age. The age will determine who is responsible for giving the consent.
   CAT: Office Operation

6. Using Black's classification of cavities, a pit lesion on the buccal of molars and premolars is considered a class _____ restoration or cavity.
   a. A class I restoration or cavity is described as a pit lesion on the buccal surface of molars and premolars using Black's classification of cavities. A class II cavity has decay that is interproximal such as mesial or distal. A class V cavity has decay on the gingival third of the facial or lingual surface. A class III cavity has decay diagnosed on the proximal surface of the anterior teeth.
   CAT: Patient Education and Oral Heath Management

7. Any tooth that remains unerupted in the jaw beyond the time at which it should normally erupt is referred to as being:
   c. An impacted tooth is one that is so positioned in the jawbone that eruption

is not possible. A fused tooth is jointed together during tooth development by one or more of the hard tissues (enamel, dentin, or cementum). Abrade refers to wearing away by friction; therefore, the tooth must be erupted. Ankylosis is an abnormal fixation and immobility of a joint and has no relationship to tooth eruption.
CAT: Patient Education and Oral Health Management

8. When assisting a right-handed operator, a preset tray is set up from:
   a. A tray is set up from left to right based on how instruments are transferred and used throughout a dental procedure. To have the instruments prepared from bottom to top would not be in a sequence of instrument transferability. From small to large is not an option for arranging instruments on a preset tray. An instrument tray is set up for the assistant to use the left hand to transfer instruments right to left is incorrect.
   CAT: Chairside Dental Procedures

9. The high-speed contra-angle handpiece reaches speed of:
   d. A high-speed operates from air pressure and reaches speeds up to 450,000 rpm. Speeds of 150,000 rpm, 250,000 and 350,000 rpm are not comparable to high speed. A low-speed handpiece is available in speeds from 10,000 to 30,000 rpm.
   CAT: Chairside Dental Procedures

10. An automated external defibrillator (AED) is used for all except to _____.
    b. The AED does not perform CPR and is basically an advanced computer that identifies any cardiac rhythm for abnormalities and, if needed, sends a massive "shock" of electricity to the heart muscle to re-establish a proper rhythm.
    CAT: Prevention and Management of Emergencies

11. _____ can be life threatening and is indicated by nausea and vomiting, shortness of breath, and loss of consciousness.
    b. Anaphylaxis is one form of a type I allergic antigen. This condition can be life threatening and is indicated by nausea and vomiting, shortness of breaths, or loss

of consciousness. Syncope is a fainting or temporary loss of consciousness caused by cerebral anemia. Low blood glucose has different symptoms such as anxiety, breath odor, and trembling. High blood pressure symptoms are blurred vision, blood in the urine, and chest pain.
CAT: Prevention and Management of Emergencies

12. The respirations of a patient who is hyperventilating will be exemplified by:
    d. A patient who is hyperventilating will display excessively long, rapid breaths. A gurgling sound involves fluid with intermitted air. Hyperventilating is not slow respirations, and neither is breathing excessively short and rapid breaths.
    CAT: Prevention and Management of Emergencies

13. The respiration pattern of a patient in a state of tachypnea has:
    c. A patient will have breaths that are excessively short and rapid. Patients with nervous tachypnea display a respiratory rate of 40 breaths/min or more. A normal respiration rate is 10 to 20 breaths/min for an adult. A gurgling sound involves fluid with intermitted air. Hyperventilation is excessively long, rapid breaths.
    CAT: Prevention and Management of Emergencies

14. The symbol on tooth #31 indicates it is:
    c. The symbol on tooth #31 indicates that it has drifted distally. The mobility of a tooth is noted on a periodontal chart with the proper rate of mobility. For a rotated tooth, the position is indicated by the directional arrow. A tooth that is drifted mesially would point in the mesial direction.
    CAT: Collection and Recording of Clinical Data

15. The symbol on tooth #8 indicates it will need to have:
    d. There is a periapical abscess on this tooth with the mesioincisal angle fractured. A periodontal treatment would not be noted at the apex of the tooth. The distoincisal edge is the opposite of the marked fracture.
    CAT: Collection and Recording of Clinical Data

16. The symbol between teeth #24 and #25 indicates:

b. The two vertical lines indicate the presence of a diastema or a space that is wider than normal between two teeth. "Heavy calculus" is written in the treatment chart to include the periodontal charting. A supernumerary tooth is represented with a diamond shape at the location of the tooth with "SN" written into the diamond. A displaced frenum attachment is written in the chart.

CAT: Collection and Recording of Clinical Data

17. The symbol on tooth #23 indicates that this tooth:

a. An implant is indicated commonly by drawing horizontal lines through the root or roots of the tooth or teeth. A root canal is a single line from the cementum enamel junction (CEJ) to the apex. A post and core is a small circle colored in and a single line in the one-third of the root of the tooth. A fractured root would have a zigzag line of the fracture.

CAT: Collection and Recording of Clinical Data

18. The symbol on tooth #3 indicates that this tooth:

a. A common symbol, S, is used to indicate the presence of a sealant. The S is indicated in red pencil to be completed. Occlusal staining is written in the treatment portion of the chart. The symbol SS is used for a stainless steel crown.

CAT: Collection and Recording of Clinical Data

19. How many permanent teeth have erupted?

b. On this chart, 10 permanent teeth have erupted—all of the permanent central incisors, the mandibular lateral incisors, and all four permanent first molars. A, C, and D are not correct because the missing teeth are marked with an "X."

CAT: Collection and Recording of Clinical Data

20. How many permanent teeth are present on the mandible?

a. All four permanent incisors are present as well as the two permanent first molars. B, C, and D are not correct because the missing teeth are marked with an "X."

CAT: Collection and Recording of Clinical Data

21. The examination technique in which the examiner uses his or her fingers and hands to feel for the size, texture, and consistency of hard and soft tissue is called:

b. Palpation is the examination technique in which the examiner uses the fingers and hands to feel for the size, texture, and consistency of hard and soft tissue. Detection is the act or process of discovering tooth imperfections or decay. Probing is using a slender, flexible instrument to explore and measure the periodontal pocket. The extraoral exam is a visual inspection of the landmarks outside the oral cavity.

CAT: Collection and Recording of Clinical Data

22. A patient's pulse rate may be decreased because of:

d. A patient taking depressants may have a decreased pulse rate. Stress causes an increase in pulse rate and blood pressure. Proper exercise and stimulants increase the pulse rate.

CAT: Collection and Recording of Clinical Data

23. Most local anesthetic agents used for dental procedures are:

d. Intermediate-acting local anesthetic agents last 120 to 240 minutes. Most local anesthetic agents are in this group and are used for dental procedures. There are many different forms of dental anesthetics. A standard dental procedure does not require a long-acting anesthetic. A short-acting anesthetic is used in combination with another or in a short procedure.

CAT: Chairside Dental Procedures

24. In the United States, nitrous oxide gas lines are color coded, _____ and oxygen lines are color coded _____.

d. In the United States, nitrous oxide gas lines are color coded blue, and oxygen gas lines are color coded green. Red tanks contain CO_2 and are not a part of a dental office. Green only indicates oxygen, and blue is nitrous. Other countries may have different color codes.

CAT: Chairside Dental Procedures

25. The dental assistant's responsibility in an emergency situation is to:
    d. The dental assistant works with the rest of the dental team to recognize the symptoms and signs of significant medical complaints and to provide appropriate support in implementing emergency procedures. A dental assistant cannot diagnose any condition at any time.
    CAT: Chairside Dental Procedures

26. A condition called _____ will result if an alginate impression absorbs additional water by being stored in water or in a very wet paper towel.
    c. Imbibition is the condition in which an alginate impression absorbs additional water, causing the impression to swell and become distorted. Alginate is a type of B hydrocolloid impression material. Syneresis is the process by which water is lost from the impression and shrinkage takes place. Polymerization is the curing reaction between two or more monomers.
    CAT: Chairside Dental Materials

27. _____ may be applied to the edge of the alginate trays to improve the fit of the tray.
    c. Utility wax is used to the edge of an alginate tray to improve the fit of a tray for definition or comfort purposes. Beading wax is used on final impressions for the tray definition. *Wax pattern* is a correct term, but *pattern wax* is not. Boxing wax is used to form a wall or box around a preliminary impression when it is poured up without the need to trim as much material.
    CAT: Chairside Dental Materials

28. The water-to-powder ratio generally used for an mandibular impression is _____ scoops of water, and _____ scoops of powder.
    d. The water-to-powder ratio used for an adult mandibular impression is generally 2 measures of water and 2 scoops of powder. The 3 measures of water to 3 measures of powder is for a maxillary impression. Measures of 4 and 3 and 2 and 4 are incorrect because if you use unequal portions of water to powder, the consistency will not set accurately.
    CAT: Chairside Dental Procedures

29. The term _____ means to move the tooth back and forth within the socket.
    b. To luxate a tooth means to move it back and forth in an attempt to dislodge it from the alveolar socket. Festoon is a carving in the base material of a denture that simulates the contours of the natural tissues being replaced by the denture. Capitation is the practice of dentistry financed by a set fee per person per given period of time. To displace (root displacement) is to remove from its normal position.
    CAT: Chairside Dental Procedures

30. _____ forceps are designed to grasp the bifurcation of the root of a mandibular molar.
    c. Cowhorn forceps have curved, pointed beaks that are designed to grasp the tooth at the furcation for easier manipulation and removal. A curved forceps is a universal term that can be considered maxillary and mandibular forceps for grasping the crown (universal mandibular or universal maxillary). The bayonet is a binangled instrument, the nib or blade of which is generally parallel to the shaft; it resembles a bayonet.
    CAT: Chairside Dental Procedures

31. When a blood clot is dislodged because of the exertion of forces such as sucking on a straw and as a result the patient experiences extreme discomfort, it is referred to as:
    c. Alveolitis occurs when the blood clot has been lost because of forces such as sucking on a straw or smoking. The patient experiences extreme pain and inflammation. Osteosis is the formation of bony tissue. Ankylosis is the fusion of bones of a joint, often as a result of disease or injury or intentionally through surgery. Acidosis is a failure of the mechanism that controls the acidity of the blood, other body fluids, or body tissues, commonly caused by untreated diabetes.
    CAT: Chairside Dental Procedures

32. The retromolar pad is reproduced in the _____ impression.
    a. The retromolar pad is slightly distal to the origin of the pterygomandibular fold

behind the last mandibular molar and is reproduced in the mandibular impression. The maxillary would not have the tongue space or the mylohyoid ridge.
CAT: Chairside Dental Procedures

33. Which of the following instruments would be used to measure the depth of the gingival sulcus?
    b. The periodontal probe is used to measure the depth of the gingival sulcus in millimeter increments. A shepherd's hook is a type of explorer that is used to detect dental caries. A cowhorn explorer, also known as a pigtail explorer, is so named because of the shape of its shank that is used to examine teeth for calculus, caries, and restoration margins. A right-angle explorer is also used to detect dental caries and not measure the depth of the sulcus but examine for calculus.
    CAT: Chairside Dental Procedures

34. Which of the following instruments has sharp, round, angular tips used to detect tooth anomalies?
    c. A cowhorn explorer is the only explorer with a rounded tip that is used to examine teeth for calculus, caries, and restoration margins. A periodontal probe is used to measure the depth of the gingival sulcus in millimeter increments. A shepherd's hook is a type of explorer that is used to detect dental caries. A right-angle explorer is also used to detect dental caries and not measure the depth of the sulcus but examine for calculus.
    CAT: Chairside Dental Procedures

35. Which instrument is commonly used to scale surfaces in the anterior region of the mouth?
    c. A straight sickle scaler is used to remove large deposits of supragingival calculus from the anterior teeth. A curet scaler is used to remove subgingival calculus and to smooth rough root surfaces and to remove the diseased soft tissue lining of the periodontal pocket. A Gracey scaler is designed to adapt to specific tooth surfaces and scale and remove deposits in deep periodontal pockets. A modified sickle scaler is a posterior scaler similar to

the straight sickle in function but with a modified shank.
    CAT: Chairside Dental Procedures

36. Which instrument is used to scale deep periodontal pockets or furcation areas?
    b. A Gracey scaler is designed to scale deep pockets and furcation areas and requires the use of several different curettes. A straight sickle scaler is used to remove large deposits of supragingival calculus from the anterior teeth. A curet scaler is used to remove subgingival calculus, smooth rough root surfaces, and remove the diseased soft tissue lining of the periodontal pocket. A modified sickle scaler is used to remove deposits of supragingival calculus from posterior teeth.
    CAT: Chairside Dental Procedures

37. In the drawing below, which area stabilizes the clamp to the tooth?
    d. Four prongs in the jaws of the clamp grasp the tooth, providing stability to the clamp when it is in place. A "winged" clamp is designed with extra extensions to help retain the dental dam. The bow is the rounded portion of the clamp that extends through the dental dam. A hole is used for the dental dam forceps to grasp the clamp and spread open the jaws around the tooth.
    CAT: Chairside Dental Procedures

38. When the operator is working in the labial of tooth #9, the HVE tip is held:
    b. By placing the HVE tip on the lingual of this tooth, the assistant will be able to efficiently remove fluids and not interfere with the operator's handpiece. On the labial surface of the tooth, the assistant would interfere with operator's field of vision. The retromolar area is in the posterior of the mouth while the tooth is an anterior tooth. The vestibule is not near the area of the tooth being treated.
    CAT: Chairside Dental Procedures

39. A right-handed dentist is doing a preparation on #30 MO. The dental assistant places the HVE tip:
    c. By placing the HVE tip on the lingual of this tooth, the assistant will be able to

efficiently remove fluids and not interfere with the operator's handpiece. On the buccal or occlusal surfaces of the tooth, the assistant blocks the view of the operator's field of vision. If placed on the buccal of #19, the tip would be on the opposite side and not efficiently pick up fluids.

CAT: Chairside Dental Procedures

40. The angle of the bevel of the HVE top should always be:
    b. By placing the HVE tip parallel to the buccal or lingual surface, the assistant is able to remove fluids from the mouth more efficiently. The angle for the bevel of the HVE should not be to the occlusal surface because the tip would obscure view of the operator. The HVE cannot be angled at right angles to the buccal and lingual surfaces because it will not effectively remove fluids from the mouth at that degree. The HVE has a proper direction in order to be effective and not interfere with the operator's vision.

    CAT: Chairside Dental Procedures

41. The cement that has a sedative effect on the pulp is known as:
    c. Zinc oxide–eugenol has a sedative effect on the pulp. Glass ionomer releases fluoride but does not protect the pulp. Zinc phosphate is the most irritating to the pulp because it is acidic. Zinc silicon phosphate is also irritating cement.

    CAT: Chairside Dental Materials (Preparation, Manipulation, and Application)

42. The wooden wedge is placed in the gingival embrasure area for Class II restorations to accomplish all *except* which of the following?
    b. The wooden wedge is not placed to adapt the band to the occlusal. The wedge does aid in preventing overhangs and a missing proximal wall as well as maintaining proximal contact for the embrasure area.

    CAT: Chairside Dental Procedures

43. Which of the following techniques could be used for caries removal?
    c. The instruments of choice would be the no. 2 RA bur and a spoon excavator because slow removal is more efficient

when removing soft carious material from a tooth. The no. 2 RA bur is the correct bur, but the enamel hatchet is used to smooth the walls of the preparation, not remove carious material. The ¼ FG bur would be too small of a bur to use to remove decay, but the spoon is correct. The no. ¼ FG bur and explorer are both incorrect because the ¼ is too small and the explorer is used for examinations not removal of decay.

CAT: Chairside Dental Procedures

44. Select the instrument that will be used to carve the distal surface of an amalgam restoration placed on 30DO.
    d. The Hollenbeck carver is a smooth surface carver and is used to carve the distal surface of an amalgam for #30. The large cleoid–discoid carver is used to carve the occlusal surface bulk of the amalgam after placement, and the smaller cleoid–discoid carver is used to carve the detailed anatomy of the occlusal surface. A scaler is not an appropriate instrument for carving an amalgam.

    CAT: Chairside Dental Materials

45. From the photograph below, select the instrument that would be used to attach to the rubber dam clamps.
    d. The dental dam forceps is the instrument that would be used to attach to the rubber dam clamp. The crown and bridge scissors are used for temporary crowns or cutting the rubber dam material. The rubber dam is placed on the patient's tooth, and the frame holds the rubber dam tightly. The rubber dam punch will punch the appropriate hole sizes into the dam for the tooth sizes and dam clamp.

    CAT: Chairside Dental Procedures

46. Which part of an anesthetic syringe differs in an aspirating and nonaspirating syringe?
    b. The harpoon is a sharp hook that locks into the rubber stopper of the anesthetic cartridge so the stopper can be retracted by pulling back on the piston rod and be able to aspirate. The syringe barrel firmly holds the anesthetic cartridge in place. The

cartridge is loaded through the open side of the barrel with an opening to watch for blood. The metal thumb ring is to control the syringe firmly and to aspirate effectively with one hand.
CAT: Chairside Dental Procedures

47. What is a contraindication for a patient using a gingival retraction cord that is impregnated with epinephrine?
    d. Epinephrine may cause problems in patients with cardiovascular conditions because it is a vasoconstrictor and has the potential to stress the heart. A patient with diabetes would have a contraindication to sugar or insulin intake. A patient with epilepsy who is prone to seizure activity may have a seizure but it would not relate to epinephrine. A patient with hypothyroidism would have issues with blood pressure changes.
    CAT: Chairside Dental Procedures

48. Which instrument would be used to check for an overhang on a newly placed restoration?
    a. The explorer, with its sharp, pointed tip, is used to examine for overhangs. A Woodson is a double-ended instrument used for carrying dental materials to the prepared tooth structure. The spoon excavator is used to remove soft dentin, debris, and decay from the tooth. The Hollenback carver is used to contour and carve occlusal and interproximal anatomy in amalgam and other restorative filling materials.
    CAT: Chairside Dental Procedures

49. Which of the following instruments would be the least likely to be used for placing a cavity liner?
    d. The amalgam condenser is the least likely to be used to place cavity liner because of the lack of control. An explorer can be used to place cavity liner in small areas. The spoon excavator can be used to place a cavity liner in most cases. The ball burnisher can be used to place the cavity liner in a tooth structure.
    CAT: Chairside Dental Procedures

50. Which of the following instruments is a Hedstrom file?
    c. A Hedstrom file is shaped like a cone with a pointed tip and triangular edges. A is a barbed broach, B is a cleoid–discoid carver, and D is an endodontic file.
    CAT: Chairside Dental Procedures

51. The purpose of acid etching a tooth when using a composite restorative is:
    c. The purpose of acid etching is to create tags on the tooth surface. The acid etch would irritate the pulp if left on too long or too close to the pulp. The dentinal tubules are sealed by varnish, not acid etchant. The formation of bond is by using a bonding agent, not an acid etchant.
    CAT: Chairside Dental Procedures

52. Which of the following would be used for smoothing the interproximal surface in a composite procedure?
    c. The finishing strip is used to smooth the interproximal surface of a composite restoration. A Hollenback carver is used to carve amalgam, not composite. The gold carving knife is used to remove flash composite material from the interproximal areas. The explorer is sharp and not able to smooth the composite but may be used to check the margins.
    CAT: Chairside Dental Procedures

53. Which endodontic instrument is used to curette the inside of the tooth to the base of the pulp chamber?
    d. The long-shank spoon is used to curette the inside of the tooth to the base of the pulp chamber to reach inside the canal. A file is used for cleaning and shaping the pulp canal. The reamer is similar in design to a file, but its cutting edges are farther apart. The explorer has a sharp, pointed tip that will not allow curettage.
    CAT: Chairside Dental Procedures

54. The indication for pit and fissure sealants is when teeth:
    a. The indication for pit and fissure sealants is when teeth are prone to caries. If teeth are not prone to caries such as large pits and fissures, then sealants are not necessary.

The only case for which sealants are needed is if there are missing areas within the sealant. The teeth that have wide fossae and are easy to clean do not need a sealant.

CAT: Chairside Dental Procedures

55. A finger rest that stabilizes the hand to lessen possibility of slipping or traumatizing the tissue in the mouth is known as a _____.
    c. The fulcrum is the finger rest that stabilizes the hand will help prevent slipping. The hinge point is a prosthetic stabilizer. The rest point is a lay term that is not correct terminology. The base is a broad term that is used in many contexts, including dental materials, but is not a term for a stabilizer or a finger rest.

    CAT: Chairside Dental Procedures

56. _____ is the form of anesthetic that renders the patient unconscious
    b. The general sedation is a form of anesthetic that places the patient in a state of unconsciousness. A local anesthetic is able to provide profound anesthesia into a specific area while the patient remains conscious. The inhalation sedation is nitrous oxide and is a relaxation gas but does to make a patient unconscious. The conscious sedation is not unconscious; therefore, the patient is awake.

    CAT: Chairside Dental Procedures

57. A tooth that has been avulsed has been:
    d. The tooth that is avulsed is knocked free from the oral cavity. The fractured tooth has a segment of the tooth missing. A tooth that is sealed with a sealant has a protective agent placed on it to protect against cavities. The restored tooth with an amalgam is a tooth that has no decay but is not avulsed.

    CAT: Chairside Dental Procedures

58. The time from when the local anesthetic takes complete effect until the complete reversal of anesthesia is the _____ of the anesthetic agent.
    a. The duration of an anesthetic is from the onset of its effectiveness until the effect is reversed. The induction is when the anesthetic is administered. Innervation

refers to the supply or distribution of nerves to a specific body part. Compression would not inhibit the time of effectiveness.

CAT: Chairside Dental Procedures

59. The lengths of the needles used in dentistry for local anesthesia administration are:
    b. The short needle is 1 inch, and the long needle is 1⅝. The ⅝- and 1-inch needles together are not appropriate lengths. The 1½- and 2-inch length needles would not work for the maxillary because the 2-inch needle is too long. The ½- and 1½-inch needles are not long enough for a mandibular block injection.

    CAT: Chairside Dental Procedures

60. The stage of anesthesia when the patient passes through excitement and becomes calm, feels no pain or sensation, and soon becomes unconscious is referred to as stage ____ of anesthesia.
    c. General anesthesia is the stage of anesthesia that begins when the patient becomes calm after stage II. Stage I or analgesia is the stage during which a patient is relaxed and fully conscious. Stage II is excitement during which the patient is less aware of his or her immediate surroundings and may start to become unconscious. Stage IV is when respiratory failure or cardiac arrest occurs when the lungs and heart slow down or stop functioning; if not reversed, the patient can die.

    CAT: Chairside Dental Procedures

61. The most common type of attachment for fixed orthodontic appliances is the:
    b. The bonded bracket is the most common type of attachment for fixed orthodontic appliances. The orthodontic band is cemented, not fixed, on the first molars of the maxillary and mandibular teeth. The arch wire is not a fixed appliance but an accessory to move the teeth. The separator is a temporary device used before orthodontic band placement.

    CAT: Chairside Dental Procedures

62. When a health contraindication is present that prevents the use of a vasoconstrictor, the retraction cord is impregnated with _____, and the cord may have a(n) _____ agent applied to it to control bleeding.

    d. For patients with cardiovascular conflicts, aluminum chloride may be used instead of epinephrine, and a hemostatic solution is used to control the bleeding. Epinephrine is contraindicated with cardiac patients. Aluminum chloride is correct, but galvanic is not a solution. Sodium chloride is a saline solution, but galvanic is not a solution.

       CAT: **Prevention and Management of Emergencies**

63. A(n) _____ is present when the maxillary teeth are positioned lingually to the mandibular teeth either unilaterally or bilaterally.

    b. A crossbite occurs when the maxillary teeth are positioned lingually to the mandibular teeth. This may be a unilateral or bilateral situation Overjet is a horizontal projection of the maxillary teeth beyond the mandibular teeth, usually measured parallel to the occlusal plane. An open bite is a malformation in which the anterior teeth do not occlude in any mandibular position. An end-to-end relationship occurs when the teeth occlude without the maxillary teeth overlapping the mandibular teeth. An end-to-end bite can occur anteriorly and posteriorly.

       CAT: **Chairside Dental Procedures**

64. What instrument is used in ligating an arch wire?

    c. A ligature tying pliers is used to tie in an arch wire with wire ligatures. A hemostat may be used but is not an ideal instrument. The Howe pliers have a flat, rounded, serrated top that allows placement and removal or creation of adjustment bends in the arch wire. The utility pliers also known as Weingart pliers, are finely serrated narrow beaks that allow accessibility to various areas. They are used in the placement of arch wires.

       CAT: **Chairside Dental Procedures**

65. A tray is set up from:

    a. A tray is set up from left to right based on how instruments are transferred and used throughout a dental procedure.

       CAT: **Chairside Dental Procedures**

66. A periodontal probe is an example of which type of instrument?

    a. A periodontal probe is an examination instrument used to measure the depth of the gingival sulcus.

       CAT: **Chairside Dental Procedures**

67. Most local anesthetic agents used for dental procedures are:

    b. Intermediate-acting local anesthetic agents last 120 to 240 minutes. Most local anesthetic agents are in this group and are used for dental procedures.

       CAT: **Chairside Dental Procedures**

68. At the correct therapeutic level, patients receiving nitrous oxide/oxygen analgesia will feel:

    c. A floating sensation is the feeling a patient will experience when he or she receives the correct therapeutic level of nitrous oxide/oxygen. Nausea, giggling, and anxiousness could be signs that the percentage of nitrous oxide versus oxygen is too high.

       CAT: **Chairside Dental Procedures**

69. Which instrument is used for interdental cutting of gingiva and to remove tissue?

    b. The Orban knife is designed for interdental cutting of gingiva and removal of tissue. The back-action hoe is used to remove bone adjacent to teeth without causing problems. The kidney-shaped periodontal knife is designed to create a bevel incision for a gingivectomy. The interdental file is designed to crush heavy calculus from interproximal areas.

       CAT: **Chairside Dental Procedures**

70. Which of the following instruments is *not* included in the basic setup for most dental procedures?

    a. The basic setup found on most dental trays includes a mouth mirror, pigtail explorer, and cotton forceps (pliers). A curette scalar is an instrument used in prophylaxis or periodontal examination and would not be included as part of the basic tray setup.

CAT: Chairside Dental Procedures

71. Which type of scaler has a rounded toe and rounded back and may be used supragingivally and subgingivally to remove fine calculus deposits?

c. The curette scaler has a rounded toe and rounded back with a semicircular working end in a cross-section. It is used to remove fine calculus from supragingival and subgingival surfaces. The sickle has a pointed toe and pointed back and removes heavy supragingival calculus deposits. The hoe and chisel have bevelled working ends and are designe to remove supragingival calculus.

CAT: Chairside Dental Procedures

72. Which instrument is used to split or section a tooth for easier removal and to reshape and recontour alveolar bone?

b. A surgical chisel is used to split or section a tooth for easier removal and to reshape and recontour alveolar bone. A rongeur is used to trim and remove excess alveolar bone after an extraction and to contour alveolar bone after single or multiple extractions. A bone file is used to remove or smooth rough edges of alveolar bone with a push–pull motion. A T-bar elevator is used on posterior teeth to loosen the tooth from the periodontal ligaments.

CAT: Chairside Dental Procedures

73. Which of the following instruments is used to trim soft tissue during an oral surgery procedure?

c. Surgical scissors are used to trim soft tissue. Suture scissors are designed to only cut suture material. A surgical curette is used after extractions to scrape the interior of the socket to remove abscesses or diseased tissue. A scalpel is used to make a precise incision into soft tissue.

CAT: Chairside Dental Procedures

74. The HVE is used to keep the mouth free of saliva, blood, debris, and water; reduce bacterial aerosol spray caused by the high-speed handpiece; and_____.

c. The HVE is used to keep the mouth free of liquid and solid debris, reduce the bacterial aerosol caused by the high-speed handpiece, and retract the patient's tongue and cheek away from the field of operation. It does not stabilize the patient or prevent dehydration of tissue. It is designed to remove water, not to rinse.

CAT: Chairside Dental Procedures

75. When the high-speed handpiece is positioned on the occlusal surface of tooth #30, where would the assistant position the HVE?

d. The dental assistant would position the HVE on the lingual surface of tooth #30 when the high-speed handpiece is positioned on the occlusal surface of this tooth. The edge of the suction tip should remain even with or slightly beyond the occlusal surface.

CAT: Chairside Dental Procedures

76. Which of the following is true about the use of cotton rolls to isolate a working area?

c. Cotton rolls must be replaced frequently during a procedure because they easily become saturated. They are easy to apply, come in a variety of sizes, and are flexible for easy adaptability inside the mouth. However, they do not provide complete isolation.

CAT: Chairside Dental Procedures

77. A wooden wedge may be used in which of the following class preparations?

c. A restoration notation of tooth #15MO indicates a proximal cavity preparation, which would require a matrix band and wooden wedge for restorative material to replace the missing proximal wall. Notations provided for teeth #31, #21, and #3 indicate either occlusal, occlusal and facial or buccal surfaces, which do not require a matrix band and wooden wedge for restoration.

CAT: Chairside Dental Procedures

78. In an instrument tray setup, which instruments are placed farthest to the right?

b. In an instrument tray, instruments are set up from left to right. The basic setup will be first (leftmost), followed by any

additional examination instruments, hand-cutting instruments, and finally restorative instruments farthest on the right.
CAT: Chairside Dental Procedures

79. Which of the photographs below illustrates an orthodontic hemostat?
   a. This orthodontic hemostat is used to hold and place materials such as separators and ligatures. This instrument has gripping and locking capabilities.
   CAT: Chairside Dental Procedures

80. Which of the following is a thermoplastic material used to stabilize an anterior clamp?
   c. Dental compound is a rigid thermoplastic impression material that can be used on a clamp to stabilize it.
   CAT: Chairside Dental Materials

81. Select two terms that describe the purpose and consistency of a dental cement used for the seating of a temporary crown.
   d. The seating of a temporary crown requires a cement base that is of luting or primary consistency, which strings for about 1 inch. The purpose of seating the crown is for temporary cementation.
   CAT: Chairside Dental Materials

82. Which type of cement must be mixed on a glass slab?
   c. Zinc phosphate cement must be mixed on a glass slab. Zinc polycarboxylate cement may be mixed on a glass slab or paper. Zinc oxide–eugenol cement can be mixed on a glass slab or on oil-resistant paper. Calcium hydroxide cement can be mixed on a glass slab or on paper.
   CAT: Chairside Dental Materials

83. Which of the following materials is recommended for polishing filled hybrid composites and resin restorations?
   b. Aluminum oxide paste is recommended for polishing filled hybrid composites and resin restorations.
   CAT: Chairside Dental Materials

84. Light curing:
   b. Light curing is used to polymerize composite resin materials and composite

resin cement. It relies on visible light because ultraviolet light was proven to be damaging to the operator's eyes. Light curing is not used to polymerize silver dental amalgam. Self-cured composites are autopolymerized. Autopolymerized composite resin materials require mixing before placement.
CAT: Chairside Dental Materials

85. The tip of the composite curing light should be held at an angle of __ degrees to the tooth.
   a. The tip of the composite curing light should be held at an angle of 90 degrees to the tooth. The depth of cure is affected by the angle of the light.
   CAT: Chairside Dental Materials

86. Composite restorative materials are usually cured for __ seconds with a halogen curing light.
   b. Composite restorative materials are usually cured for 20 seconds with a halogen curing light. Some newer, high-intensity lights cure composite restorative material in less time. Composite core material is usually cured for 60 seconds. It is always important to follow the manufacturer's recommendations regarding curing time.
   CAT: Chairside Dental Materials

87. Hardness of a material is ranked using the:
   c. The hardness of a material is ranked using the Moh scale.
   CAT: Lab Materials and Procedures

88. Addition of very warm water to an alginate mix will cause the setting time to be:
   b. When warm water is added to an alginate mix, the material will set faster; thus, the setting time is decreased.
   CAT: Lab Materials and Procedures

89. A negative reproduction of the patient's dental arch is referred to as a(n):
   d. An impression is a negative reproduction of the patient's dental arch. When this impression is poured with a gypsum product, the end result will be a positive reproduction of the dental arch.
   CAT: Lab Materials and Procedures

90. The impression automix system can be used for all but which of the following?

d. A putty wash system is prepared in a totally different process than the syringe tray technique for which the automix system has been designed.
CAT: Lab Materials and Procedures

91. The process by which the resin material is changed from a pliable state to a hardened restoration is known as:
a. A light-cured material does not harden until it has been exposed to a curing light. This allows a more flexible working time.
CAT: Lab Materials and Procedures

92. The RDAs are the levels of essential nutrients that are needed by individuals on a daily basis. RDA stands for:
a. The Food and Nutrition Board of the National Academy of Sciences has determined the RDA levels of essential nutrients that are needed by individuals on a daily basis. These are referred to as the recommended dietary allowances.
CAT: Patient Education and Oral Health Management

93. The only nutrients that can build and repair body tissues are:
a. The primary function of proteins is to build and repair body tissues.
CAT: Patient Education and Oral Health Management

94. _____ can prevent cholesterol from oxidizing and damaging arteries.
d. In addition to lowering the dietary intake of cholesterol, increasing the intake of antioxidants may be beneficial. Antioxidant vitamins are A and E and beta-carotene. Many fruits and vegetables also contain naturally occurring antioxidants.
CAT: Patient Education and Oral Health Management

95. A patient is to take a medication three times a day. The prescription will indicate to the pharmacy that it is taken:
b. The Latin *ter in die* (tid) means "three times a day."
CAT: Patient Education and Oral Health Management

96. If the signature line on a prescription states 1 tab QID prn pain, it indicates that the patient would take the medication:
c. The Latin *quater in die* means "four times a day," and prn means *pro re nata* "as circumstances may require or as necessary." Thus, the patient is directed to take one tablet four times a day as needed for pain.
CAT: Patient Education and Oral Health Management

97. The eating disorder that can easily be recognized in the dental office by severe wear on the lingual surface of the teeth caused by stomach acid from repeated vomiting is:
a. Bulimia is an eating disorder that is characterized by binge eating and self-induced vomiting. The stomach acid from vomiting results in severe wear on the lingual surface of the teeth.
CAT: Patient Education and Oral Health Management

98. Inflammation of the supporting tissues of the teeth that begins with _____ can progress into the connective tissue and alveolar bone that supports the teeth and become _____.
c. Gingivitis is the first stage of periodontitis. Unless this condition is arrested, the inflammation progresses into the periodontium and develops into periodontitis.
CAT: Patient Education and Oral Health Management

99. MyPyramid, formerly known as the Food Guide Pyramid, is an outline of what to eat each day. The food group represented by the second smallest section on the pyramid is:
b. The second smallest food group segment on MyPyramid is meat and beans. The widths are a general guide, not exact proportions.
CAT: Patient Education and Oral Health Management

100. _____ are found mainly in fruits, grains, and vegetables, and _____ are found in processed foods such as jelly, bread, crackers, and cookies.

c. Whereas complex carbohydrates are found mainly in fruits, grains, and vegetables, simple sugars are found in processed foods such as donuts, jelly, bread, and cookies. Simple sugars are absorbed first; the complex sugars must be processed before they can be absorbed into the intestinal tract.
CAT: Patient Education and Oral Health Management

101. Subgingival calculus occurs _____ the gingival margin and can be _____ in color because of subgingival bleeding.
   d. Subgingival calculus forms on root surfaces below the gingival margin and can extend into the periodontal pockets. It can be dark green or black.
   CAT: Patient Education and Oral Health Management

102. The "A" in the ABCDs of basic life support stands for:
   c. In all emergency situations, the rescuers must promptly initiate the ABCDs of basic life support: airway, breathing, circulation, and defibrillation.
   CAT: Patient Education and Oral Health Management

103. A patient who displays symptoms of intermittent blinking, mouth movements, a blank stare, and nonresponsiveness to surroundings may be displaying symptoms of:
   a. Common symptoms of a petit mal seizure are intermittent blinking, mouth movements, a blank stare, and being not responsive to surroundings. This condition does not result in loss of consciousness, as does a grand mal seizure.
   CAT: Patient Education and Oral Health Management

104. In which of the following procedures could the patient be placed in an upright position?
   d. Although it is a procedure that could be done in a supine position, most operators prefer to take diagnostic impressions in an upright position to avoid any problems with the impression materials going into the throat area.
   CAT: Patient Education and Oral Health Management

105. Supragingival calculus is found on the _____ of the teeth above the margin of the _____.
   c. Whereas the clinical crown is the portion of the tooth that is visible in the oral cavity, the anatomic crown is the portion of the tooth that is covered with enamel. Supragingival calculus forms on the clinical crowns of the teeth above the gingiva.
   CAT: Patient Education and Oral Health Management

106. Subgingival calculus occurs _____ the gingival margin and can be _____ in color because of subgingival bleeding.
   c. Subgingival calculus forms below the gumline and may be black because of bleeding tissue.
   CAT: Patient Education and Oral Health Management

107. The most common indication for placing pit and fissure sealants would include which of the following tooth characteristics?
   d. Posterior teeth, especially newly erupted, with deep pits and fissures are ideal for sealants.
   CAT: Patient Education and Oral Health Management

108. What step(s) should the dental assistant take before applying topical fluoride?
   c. Before placing fluoride trays, the teeth should be dried to allow for maximum uptake.
   CAT: Patient Education and Oral Health Management

109. Which microorganism must be present for caries formation to begin?
   d. *Streptococcus mutans* is one of the primary factors for the formation of dental caries.
   CAT: Patient Education and Oral Health Management

110. Which energy nutrients come from plant sources?
   a. Carbohydrates, especially good ones from plant sources, are primary sources of energy.
   CAT: Patient Education and Oral Health Management

111. A patient has the following amalgam restorations: 29MO, 30^{MOD}, 31DO, and 32°.

The fee for each surface is $115. What is the fee for services rendered?

d. The per surface fee is multiplied by the number of surfaces restored. In this case, eight surfaces were restored. The total fee for this appointment is $920.
CAT: Office Operations

112. Consent is:
    b. Consent is a voluntary acceptance or agreement to what is planned or done by another person. Consent is given freely by the patient.
    CAT: Office Operations

113. A dentist retires to another state and closes the practice. The entire staff is released from employment, and the records remain in the office, but the patients are not notified of the dentist's retirement. Failure to notify the patients of the changes in the practice is called:
    b. A dentist has an obligation to inform the patients of any change in the practice ownership. If the dentist fails to notify the patients of the changes in the practice, the dentist is guilty of abandoning the patients.
    CAT: Office Operations

114. Which of the following is *not* a component of a clinical record?
    d. The recall card is a separate record or database from the clinical chart. It is based on this record or database that patients are notified of their next recall visit.
    CAT: Office Operations

115. Which of the following records is considered a vital record?
    a. Records are categorized according to their importance in the office. The patient's clinical chart is considered a vital record; without its availability, the patient history and treatment would not be available.
    CAT: Office Operations

116. Which member of the dental team is legally required to report suspected child abuse?

b. The dentist is the only member of the dental team legally required to report suspected child abuse, although all members of the team have a moral responsibility to report suspected abuse to the dentist.
CAT: Office Operations

117. A dentist informs you that a patient will need three appointments to complete a three-unit bridge. These appointments will likely to be:
    a. The appointment schedule to seat a bridge includes the preparation, the try on of the components, and then the final cementation appointment.
    CAT: Office Operations

118. An administrative assistant has failed to maintain the recall system for the past 4 months. Which is likely to occur?
    a. The recall system is the lifeline of the practice. If patients are not routinely recalled to the dental office for preventive prophylaxis, the lack of follow-up treatment will cause decreased productivity.
    CAT: Office Operations

119. After a routine examination and prophylaxis of a 19-year-old female patient, the doctor diagnoses three restorations; the patient's mother calls to discuss her daughter's treatment plan. You politely and respectfully:
    c. Because the patient is a legal adult, written consent must be obtained directly from the patient before any discussion occurs.
    CAT: Office Operations

120. A dental assistant orders supplies once per week and has been instructed to always maintain a 30-day supply of materials in the practice. The supply of syringes of composite shade A has been depleted and the practice uses these at a rate of one tube every 15 days. How many syringes should be ordered?
    b. The assistant will order two syringes to maintain the inventory at 30 days.
    CAT: Office Operations

Radiation Health and Safety

1. Which of the following contribute to an underexposed image?
   d. An underexposed image results from inadequate exposure time. Other reasons for an underexposed image include inadequate mA or kVp settings.
   CAT: Expose and Evaluate: Evaluate

2. Intensifying screens would be used with which of the following films?
   d. Intensifying screens are held in the panoramic cassette with the film between them. Screen film is used in panoramic imaging and is sensitive to the light emitted from intensifying screens. No such screens are found in any of the other types of film.
   CAT: Radiation Safety for Patients and Operators

3. Which is the true statement concerning the anode?
   d. The tungsten target in the anode converts bombarding electrons into x-ray photons. The anode carries a positive charge, electrons are generated at the cathode, and the cathode consists of a tungsten filament in a focusing cup.
   CAT: Radiation Safety for Patients and Operators

4. During the production of x-rays, how much energy is lost as heat?
   d. Electrons travel from the cathode to the anode. When the electrons strike the tungsten target, their energy of motion or kinetic energy is converted to x-ray energy and heat. Less than 1% of the energy is converted to x-rays. X-ray production is very inefficient; 99% of the energy used to generate x-rays is lost as heat.
   CAT: Radiation Safety for Patients and Operators

5. If the length of the PID is changed from 8 to 16 inches, how does this affect the intensity of the x-ray beam?
   b. Using the Inverse Square Law, the correct answer is the beam would be one-quarter as intense. The Inverse Square Law states that "the intensity of radiation is inversely proportional to the square of the distance from the source of radiation."
   CAT: Radiation Safety for Patients and Operators

6. What is the effect on a film if the exposure time was decreased?
   c. If the exposure time is decreased, the density decreases and the image appears lighter. If the exposure time is decreased, less x-rays reach the receptor and the radiograph appears light.
   CAT: Radiation Safety for Patients and Operators

7. What is the type of contrast desirable when looking for periodontal disease?
   b. Because periodontal disease may appear as slight changes in the bone, an image with low contrast has many shades of gray and is useful for the detection of periodontal disease. An image with high contrast has many black and white areas and is useful for the detection of dental caries.
   CAT: Expose and Evaluate: Evaluate

8. What landmark is circled on the radiograph?
   b. This is the lingual foramen. It is an opening or a hole in the bone located on the internal surface of the mandible near the midline; it is surrounded by the genial tubercles and appears radiolucent.
   CAT: Expose and Evaluate: Evaluate

9. Which of the following pieces of equipment requires heat sterilization before use?
   d. Beam alignment devices must be packaged in sterilized bags and dispensed from a central supply area. Dental film, digital sensors, and the x-ray tubehead are not heat sterilized.
   CAT: Infection Control: Standard Precautions for Equipment

10. What landmark is indicated by the arrows?
    c. The radiolucent area in this image is the floor of the maxillary sinus, which is one of a paired cavity or compartment of bone located within the maxilla.
    CAT: Expose and Evaluate: Evaluate

11. Which type of film is used in panoramic radiography?
    a. Screen film is used in panoramic radiography. This type of film is sensitive to the light that is emitted from the intensifying screens.
    CAT: Expose and Evaluate: Assessment and Preparation

12. Which statement is NOT correct concerning the exposure sequence for periapical images?
    b. The dental radiographer should always have an established exposure routine to prevent errors and use the time most efficiently. Failure to do this may result in omitting an area or exposing it twice. Routinely, when using the paralleling technique for periapical images, always start with the anterior teeth first on the maxillary and then on the mandible. When working from the right to the left in the maxillary arch and then left to right in the mandibular arch, no wasted movement or shifting of the position-indicating device (PID) occurs. After anterior images are exposed, the premolar and molar images can be exposed, again using an efficient system of placement.
    CAT: Expose and Evaluate: Acquire

13. Which of the following conditions exists on this image?
    b. This view indicates open contacts between the maxillary premolars as evidenced by the dark spaces between these teeth.
    CAT: Expose and Evaluate: Evaluate

14. What is the appearance of the processing error termed "reticulation"?
    c. Reticulation of emulsion causes the film to appear cracked. A network of corrugations in the film emulsion gives it this cracked appearance. A processing error that causes the film to be black is overdevelopment. Underdeveloped film will be lighter. Yellow-brown stains can be caused by

exhausted developer or fixer or insufficient fixing or rinsing.
    CAT: Expose and Evaluate: Evaluate

15. Label the solutions used in an automatic film processor from left to right.
    b. From left to right, the solutions in an automatic film processor are (1) developing solution, (2) fixing solution, and (3) water wash.
    CAT: Expose and Evaluate: Acquire

16. What is the purpose of including a lead collimator inside the dental tubehead?
    b. The collimator restricts the size and shape of the x-ray beam as it exits the tubehead. The lead plate reduces the surface area exposed by x-radiation.
    CAT: Radiation Safety for Patients and Operators

17. What is the term to describe the point in radiation exposure when cell death occurs?
    b. The period of injury occurs where many injuries may result, including cell death. After the latent period, a period of injury occurs.
    CAT: Radiation Safety for Patients and Operators

18. Which radiology item is replaced by a digital sensor?
    c. In digital radiography, the sensor is a small detector that is placed intraorally to capture a radiographic image, thus replacing intraoral dental film.
    CAT: Expose and Evaluate: Acquire

19. When exposing intraoral radiographs, in which the patient's right is on your left, the identification dot on the film will be positioned where?
    a. When the raised side of the identification dot is facing the viewer, the radiographs are then being viewed from the labial aspect. The patient's left side is on the viewer's right, and the patient's right side is on the viewer's left side as if the viewer is looking directly at the patient. The dot should be directed toward the incisal edge or occlusal surface to not be a part of the diagnostic area.
    CAT: Expose and Evaluate: Acquire

20. In which two lengths are PIDs typically available?

 c. Position-indicating devices or cones appear as an extension of the x-ray tubehead and are used to direct the x-ray beam. They are typically available in two lengths: short (8 inches) and long (16 inches).
  CAT: Expose and Evaluate: Acquire

21. How should the film be placed when exposing a mandibular occlusal radiograph?

 b. To expose an occlusal film, the film is placed between the occlusal surfaces of both arches with the white side facing the arch that is being exposed.
  CAT: Expose and Evaluate: Acquire

22. Direct digital imaging involves digitizing an existing x-ray film using a CCD camera. Indirect digital imaging is superior to direct digital imaging.

 b. Indirect digital imaging is the method of obtaining a digital image in which an existing radiograph is scanned and converted into a digital form using a CCD camera. This method does not provide the same quality as would direct imaging.
  CAT: Expose and Evaluate: Acquire

23. Which of the following refers to operator protection during radiographic procedures?

 a. The operator should avoid the primary beam. The use of a lead apron and practice of avoiding retakes protect the patient. Determining the need for radiographs is the responsibility of the dentist.
  CAT: Radiation Safety for Patients and Operators

24. Which landmark would be found in the mandibular molar exposure?

 d. The external oblique ridge is seen in the mandibular molar exposure.
  CAT: Expose and Evaluate: Assessment and Preparation

25. Which form of radiation is found in the environment and includes cosmic and terrestrial radiation?

 d. Background radiation comes from natural sources such as radioactive materials in the ground and cosmic radiation from space.
  CAT: Radiation Safety for Patients and Operators

26. Which of the following statements is TRUE as it relates to the direct theory of radiation?

 a. The direct theory of radiation injury suggests that cell damage results when ionizing radiation directly hits critical areas or targets within the cell. This occurs when the x-ray photon directly strikes the DNA within the cell, resulting in injury to the irradiated organism.
  CAT: Radiation Safety for Patients and Operators

27. Which cells are affected when radiation exposure produces mutations to future generations?

 c. Radiation exposure to genetic cells could produce mutations in a future generation.
  CAT: Radiation Safety for Patients and Operators

28. Which body tissue listed is the most sensitive to radiation exposure?

 b. Of the body tissues listed, bone marrow is the most sensitive to radiation exposure.
  CAT: Radiation Safety for Patients and Operators

29. When converting to digital radiography, which aspect of the process remains a concern for dental offices?

 a. Even though the amount of radiation generated while exposing digital images is reduced by as much as 60%, radiation is still cumulative and a lead apron should always be used on the patient.
  CAT: Expose and Evaluate: Assessment and Preparation

30. Which exposure method would produce the smallest patient dose of radiation?

 d. Although F-speed film reduces the patient dose by approximately 60% over E-speed film, the smallest dose of radiation will occur using a digital sensor. There is no G-speed film at this time.
  CAT: Radiation Safety for Patients and Operators

31. A bite-wing image shows the _____ of both the _____ and _____.
    c. A bite-wing image shows the crowns of both the maxilla and the mandible.
       CAT: Expose and Evaluate: Assessment and Preparation

32. The collimator:
    b. The collimator is a diaphragm, usually lead, used to restrict the size and shape of the x-ray beam.
       CAT: Radiation Safety for Patients and Operators

33. After a lead apron is used, it should be:
    d. After a lead apron has been used, it must be disinfected and hung up or laid on a rounded bar. It should never be folded because it will crack, and permanent damage will make it ineffective.
       CAT: Radiation Safety for Patients and Operators

34. The _____ image provides a wide view of the maxilla and mandible.
    c. The panoramic image is an extraoral radiograph that is designed to provide a wide view of the maxilla and mandible on a single image.
       CAT: Expose and Evaluate: Assessment and Preparation

35. _____ film can be used in cassettes.
    c. An extraoral radiographic examination provides inspection of large areas of the skull or jaws using film placed in a cassette outside the mouth. The cassette is a light-tight device that holds the film and intensifying screens.
       CAT: Expose and Evaluate: Assessment and Preparation

36. To increase the contrast on a radiograph, one should _____ the kilovoltage peak.
    a. Contrast refers to how sharply dark and light areas are differentiated or separated on a film. When low kilovoltage peak settings are used, a high-contrast image will result.
       CAT: Radiation Safety for Patients and Operators

37. A tissue that lies within the primary dental beam and is very radio-sensitive is the _____.
    b. When evaluating the effects of radiation on tissues and organs, the cornea is considered a high-sensitivity organ.
       CAT: Radiation Safety for Patients and Operators

38. A _____ radiograph provides a view that shows the tooth crown, root tip, and surrounding structures of a specific area.
    b. A periapical radiograph provides a view that shows the tooth crown, root tip, and surrounding structures of a specific area and is widely used in diagnostic procedures.
       CAT: Expose and Evaluate: Assessment and Preparation

39. In a dental practice in which many HIV-positive patients are treated, the film rollers in the automatic processor should be _____.
    d. Using Standard Precautions, all processing equipment is maintained in the usual accepted manner for all patients.
       CAT: Infection Control: Standard Precautions for Equipment

40. _____ is an example of a patient protection technique used before x-ray exposure.
    b. Proper prescribing of radiographs is an example of a patient protection technique because it limits the patient's exposure to radiation. The professional judgment of the dentist is used to determine the number, type, and frequency of dental radiographs. Every patient's dental condition is different; therefore, every patient must be evaluated for dental radiographs on an individual basis.
       CAT: Radiation Safety for Patients and Operators

41. Inherent filtration in the dental x-ray tubehead: _____.
    a. Inherent filtration takes place when the primary beam passes through the glass window of the x-ray tube, the insulating oil, and the tubehead seal. Inherent filtration alone does not meet the

standards regulated by state and federal law. Therefore, added filtration is required.
CAT: Radiation Safety for Patients and Operators

42. Before radiation exposure for a minor, informed consent _____.
    b. Consent for radiographs must be obtained from a parent or legal guardian. Legally, it cannot be obtained from another person.
    CAT: Radiation Safety for Patients and Operators

43. Rules of radiation protection for the operator include all of the following EXCEPT _____.
    c. Distance recommendations indicate that the radiographer must stand at least 6 feet away from the x-ray tubehead during x-ray exposure or a protective barrier must be used.
    CAT: Radiation Safety for Patients and Operators

44. Personnel monitoring of radiation exposure _____.
    b. The amount of x-radiation that reaches the body of the dental radiographer can be measured through the use of a personnel-monitoring device known as a *film badge*. The radiographer wears it for a specified time, and the badge is returned to the service company, which in turn provides to the dental office an exposure report for each radiographer.
    CAT: Radiation Safety for Patients and Operators

45. The acronym for the permitted lifetime accumulated dose is _____.
    c. The maximum accumulated dose (MAD) is the maximum radiation dose that may be received by persons who are occupationally exposed to radiation.
    CAT: Radiation Safety for Patients and Operators

46. To prevent occupational exposure to radiation, which is the most critical for a dental radiographer?

d. Safe practice during radiographic exposure first requires that the radiographer avoid exposure to the primary beam.
CAT: Radiation Safety for Patients and Operators

47. All of the following relate to operator safety EXCEPT _____.
    d. The paralleling technique is a patient protection. All of the other answers relate to operator protection.
    CAT: Radiation Safety for Patients and Operators

48. From which of the following metals is the filter made?
    d. The filter is made of aluminum, the collimator is made of lead, the copper stem draws off the heat from the target, and the target and focal spot on the anode are made of tungsten.
    CAT: Radiation Safety for Patients and Operators

49. Thermionic emission occurs at the filament on the cathode and is controlled by the:
    a. The mA circuitry controls the heating of the filament and thermionic emission, and the kVp setting controls the speed of the electrons from the cathode to the anode. The focal spot is on the anode, and the exposure button controls how long x-ray energy is produced.
    CAT: Radiation Safety for Patients and Operators

50. An increase in exposure time will result in a radiograph that is:
    a. Increasing exposure time will result in an increase in overall darkness or density. Conversely, a decrease in exposure time will result in a lighter film.
    CAT: Radiation Safety for Patients and Operators

51. Which of the following prevents further penetration of the primary beam?
    c. The lead foil in the film packet absorbs the remainder of the primary beam, preventing further penetration into the oral cavity The x-ray energy can penetrate the vinyl

packet and the black paper surrounding the film. A cassette does not prevent panoramic film from receiving x-ray energy, and the intensifying screen in a panoramic cassette does not prevent the film from receiving x-ray energy.
CAT: **Radiation Safety for Patients and Operators**

52. Which of the following is a true statement regarding radiation and patient protection?
   d. The benefit of early diagnosis of dental disease far outweighs the risks related to ionizing radiation. Exposure of radiographs is based on clinical need and not based on a "time" routine. Rectangular collimators reduce the area of exposure on the face more than round collimators. At no time should a patient hold a film in place.
   CAT: **Radiation Safety for Patients and Operators**

53. Which of the following methods is LEAST effective in helping a patient understand the value of dental radiographs?
   c. Allowing a patient to observe another patient in treatment would not only be inappropriate, but would add little to an understanding of the value of a dental radiographic examination. Providing literature and education through discussion with the dentist would be considered an appropriate and responsible approach.
   CAT: **Expose and Evaluate: Patient Management**

54. Who determines the number, type, and frequency of dental radiographs?
   d. The guidelines for dental radiographic procedures are determined by the ADA, not the professional staff.
   CAT: **Expose and Evaluate: Patient Management**

55. When a patient who refuses to have dental radiographs taken offers to sign a waiver of responsibility, what is the most appropriate action?
   a. A patient cannot sign away his/her rights to care. Signing a waiver of refusal of treatment does not obviate professional responsibility.
   CAT: **Expose and Evaluate: Patient Management**

56. Areas in the oral cavity most likely to cause a gag reflex when stimulated include the _____.
   a. The soft palate and lateral borders of the tongue are trigger points of a gag response. The floor of the mouth, posterior of the tongue, hard palate, and palatoglossal arch do not contain the sensory nerve ending that would trigger a gag reflex.
   CAT: **Expose and Evaluate: Patient Management**

57. Proper film size for an edentulous patient is_____.
   c. Size 2 film is most appropriate for use in an edentulous area or mouth; it is the standard film used to examine all areas of the mouth. Size 1 is used to examine anterior teeth in adults. Size 0 film is the smallest and used to examine posterior teeth in small children. Size 3 is longer and narrower and is used for bite-wing images. Some digital radiography sensors also come in sizes to mimic those of film.
   CAT: **Expose and Evaluate: Patient Management**

58. Which of the following describes one reason for the difficulty encountered in trying to expose an image of a tooth undergoing an endodontic procedure?
   c. The equipment required for an endodontic procedure – the rubber dam and housing – creates obstacles to producing a dental radiograph.
   CAT: **Expose and Evaluate: Patient Management**

59. Proper handling of replenisher solution includes:
   _____.
   a. Replenishing both fixer and developer will ensure properly developed images; the specific amount is determined by the frequency of use.
   CAT: **Quality Assurance**

60. Which of the following are ideal temperature and humidity levels for film storage?
   a. Film should not be stored below 50 degrees F or 25% humidity or above 70 degrees F or 50% humidity.
   CAT: **Quality Assurance**

61. The hardening agent in fixer solution is

_____.

b. Potassium alum is the hardening agent in a fixer solution. Acetic acid is an acidifier; sodium sulfite is a preservative in the developer solution; thiosulfate is a fixing agent.

CAT: Quality Assurance

62. The GBX-2 safelight filter by Kodak is considered appropriate to develop which of the following types of films?

c. Both intraoral and extraoral films are processed under the same safelight conditions.

CAT: Quality Assurance

63. Thermometers for manual processing should be placed in the _____.

a. The developing time is directly affected by temperature. Thermometers are kept in the developer tank in a manual processing system.

CAT: Quality Assurance

64. Residual gelatin and dirt can be removed from the rollers of the automatic processor with which of the following?

a. The rollers of an automatic processor need to be cleaned regularly due to a residual gelatin buildup. A cleaning film can be used to safely remove the buildup. Chemicals and cloths can damage the rollers.

CAT: Quality Assurance

65. Which of the following does not affect the life of processing solutions?

c. The life of processing solutions are affected by the number of films being processed, the care in solution preparation, and the age of the solutions. The type of safelight used in processing does not affect the life of processing solutions.

CAT: Quality Assurance

66. Automatic film processing has the following advantages over manual film processing EXCEPT which of the following?

b. Automatic processors save time, can accept films from several patients at one time, and require less maintenance than manual processing systems. The quality of the

resulting x-ray images, however, is not an advantage.

CAT: Quality Assurance

67. The purpose of the stirring rod in a manual processing tank is to

_____.

d. The stirring rod in a manual tank agitates the chemicals and equalizes the temperature in the tanks. It is used in all the tanks, not just the developer, wash, or fixer.

CAT: Quality Assurance

68. A film duplicator is a _____.

b. Duplicate films are made using a special light source, not radiation or a print process; they are duplicated under specific conditions.

CAT: Radiology Regulations

69. When placing duplicating film over the arranged radiographs, in which direction is the emulsion is placed?

b. The duplication film must be placed emulsion-side-down over the arranged radiographs.

CAT: Radiology Regulations

70. Unused developer solution may be considered hazardous because _____.

d. Unused developer has a high pH and is considered hazardous.

CAT: Radiology Regulations

71. Silver recovered from used fixer and rinse water solutions must be disposed of by which of the following means?

c. Silver recovered from fixer solution must be picked up and disposed of by an appropriate waste management service. It cannot be discharged in the sanitary sewer, septic tank, or biohazard bag.

CAT: Radiology Regulations

72. Designing and seeing to it that a hazard communication plan is in place and properly adhered to is the responsibility of

_____.

d. The employer, not the staff, is responsible for designing, putting into place, and enforcing a hazard communication plan.

CAT: Radiology Regulations

73. The term MSDS (material safety data sheets) is being replaced by which of the following terms?

d. The new term for date sheets containing safety information is Safety Data Sheets (SDS).

CAT: Radiology Regulations

74. Which type of material can cause irritating skin, eyes, or lungs and can cause illness or death?

a. Toxic materials are irritating to the skin, eyes, or lungs and can cause illness or death. An infectious material can transmit germs or certain diseases. Reactive materials can burn or explode when mixed with other materials such as air, water, or heat. Ignitable materials can ignite or burn easily.

CAT: Radiology Regulations

75. The Hazardous Communication Standard is sometimes also called _____.

b. The Employee Right to Know Standard is a synonym of The Hazardous Communication Standard.

CAT: Radiology Regulations

76. According to GHS, all chemicals will contain the following information EXCEPT which of the following?

d. All chemicals must contain the signal word, pictogram, and hazard statement, but the date of manufacture is not a requirement.

CAT: Radiology Regulations

77. Repair of dental radiography equipment is done by which of the following?

a. A properly qualified service technician would be involved in the repair of dental radiography equipment. The dentist and staff members are not usually qualified.

CAT: Radiology Regulations

78. Following processing, fresh and properly stored film will appear _____.

a. Properly stored fresh dental films will appear clear with a slight blue tint. If they appear foggy, totally black, our cloudy, a storage or processing error needs to be identified.

CAT: Radiology Regulations

79. Testing the safelight should be done at which frequency?

b. Testing the safelight should be done twice annually to ensure quality control of radiographic processes.

CAT: Radiology Regulations

80. EPA-registered chemical germicides labeled as *sterilants* are classified as

_____.

a. EPA-registered chemical germicides labeled as a *sterilants* are classified as high-level disinfectants. EPA-registered chemical germicides labeled as *tuberculocidal* are classified as intermediate-level disinfectants. EPA-registered chemical germicides labeled as *hospital disinfectants* are classified as low-level disinfectants.

CAT: Infection Control: Standard Precautions for Equipment

81. Following an exposure, beam alignment devices are placed for processing by _____ hands.

a. Beam alignment devices are contaminated with saliva; they need to be placed for processing by a gloved hand.

CAT: Infection Control: Standard Precautions for Equipment

82. Which describes the level of disinfectant appropriate for disinfection of a sensor?

b. As a semicritical instrument, a sensor should be disinfected with an intermediate-level disinfectant.

CAT: Infection Control: Standard Precautions for Equipment

83. Where in the dental practice would a list of all the chemicals used in the processing of dental films be found?

c. The written Hazard Communication Plan lists all the chemical used in the processing of dental films. An employee handbook organizes the policies and procedures of a specific practice. Engineering controls address the protocols needed to comply with regulations of safety. The Bloodborne Pathogen Standard covers infection control issues.

CAT: Infection Control: Standard Precautions for Equipment

84. Safety data sheets have _____ sections.
    d. The 16 sections of an SDS are identification, hazards identification, composition, first-aid measures, firefighting measures, accidental release measures, handling and storage, exposure controls/personal protection, physical and chemical properties, stability and reactivity, toxicological information, ecological information, disposal considerations, transport information, regulatory information, and other information.
    CAT: Infection Control: Standard Precautions for Equipment

85. Which is the method used to prevent cross-contamination during use of a digital sensor?
    e. The use of a digital sensor involves disinfection and barrier technique protocols.
    CAT: Infection Control: Standard Precautions for Equipment

86. Infection control practiced during exposure involves all of the following EXCEPT _____.
    a. The disposal of all contaminated items occurs at the end of the exposure process, not during it.
    CAT: Infection Control: Standard Precautions for Equipment

87. Washing with an alcohol-based product until hands are dry describes which term?
    b. An antiseptic hand rub is an alcohol-based product useful in dentistry when soap and water are not available.
    CAT: Infection Control: Standard Precautions for Patient and Operators

88. An instrument that contacts mucous membranes but does not penetrate soft tissue or bone is considered _____.
    b. An instrument that contacts mucous membranes but does not penetrate soft tissue or bone is considered a semicritical instrument. An instrument that contacts mucous membranes and penetrates soft tissue or bone is considered a critical instrument. An instrument that does not contact mucous membranes is considered a noncritical instrument.
    CAT: Infection Control: Standard Precautions for Patient and Operators

89. Which procedure must be performed before gloving?
    d. Before the beam alignment device is prepared, headrest adjustments and placement of the lead apron should be done with ungloved hands.
    CAT: Infection Control: Standard Precautions for Patient and Operators

90. Which choice describes recommended protocol for asking a parent to assist with an uncooperative child?
    c. The parent should hold the child in his/her lap, and both the patient and the child must be protected from scatter radiation.
    CAT: Infection Control: Standard Precautions for Patient and Operators

91. Which choice describes a single-use item in a radiographic procedure?
    b. The patient chart, beam alignment devices, and film mounts are all nondisposable items used in a radiographic procedure. Cotton rolls are single-use items that should be disposed of after a single use.
    CAT: Infection Control: Standard Precautions for Patient and Operators

92. Examples of items to clean, disinfect, and/or protect with surface barriers in dental radiography are:_____.
    e. Beam alignment devices are not disinfected and protected by barriers; infection control practices for the tubehead and exposure panel include disinfection and barrier protection.
    CAT: Infection Control: Standard Precautions for Patient and Operators

93. Which is the first step in handling film with barrier envelopes during processing?
    d. Once films are transported for processing, a towel is placed next to the transport receptacle on the work surface. Barriers are removed with gloved hands.
    CAT: Infection Control: Standard Precautions for Patient and Operators

94. In a dental radiographic procedure, which is the LEAST likely mode of disease transmission?
    d. In a dental radiographic procedure, contamination can possibly occur from airborne particles, indirect transmission, and blood but not from sexual transmission.
    CAT: Infection Control: Standard Precautions for Patient and Operators

95. The greatest infection control risk of the dental professional in radiographic procedures is from _____.
    b. Exposing, fixing, and mounting dental radiographs do not pose an infection control risk to the operator. Handling exposed dental films, however, exposes the dental professional to contaminants.
    CAT: Infection Control: Standard Precautions for Patient and Operators

96. When dental films not in barrier sleeves are exposed and removed from the oral cavity, they are _____.
    c. Dental x-ray films are never placed in a pocket, dropped on the counter, or placed into a transfer container without first being wiped.
    CAT: Infection Control: Standard Precautions for Patient and Operators

97. Film holders should be
    _____.

    e. Film holders should not be placed in a patient's chart or disinfected. They need to be heat-tolerant for sterilization, or disposable.
    CAT: Infection Control: Standard Precautions for Patient and Operators

98. Which describes appropriate protocol for single-use devices in a radiography procedure?
    b. Single-use does not mean multiple-use. The item should be discarded after use and cannot be used again.
    CAT: Infection Control: Standard Precautions for Patient and Operators

99. How must the counter and or work area be prepared before the patient is seated?
    e. Prior to seating a patient for a dental radiographic procedure, the surface must be disinfected and protected with a barrier. Disinfecting a surface alone is not thorough enough for infection control.
    CAT: Infection Control: Standard Precautions for Patient and Operators

100. In this panoramic radiograph, which of the following statements is TRUE?
    c. From this radiograph, it is evident that the permanent maxillary canines are malpositioned.

    CAT: Expose and Evaluate: Evaluate

Infection Control

1. If you opt not to receive a hepatitis B vaccination, you will be required to sign:
    c. If an employee initially declines the vaccination but at a later date opts to have the vaccine and is still covered under the standard, the employer must provide the vaccine at no cost to the employee. A copy of this informed refusal is kept on file in the dental office.
    CAT: Patient and Dental Healthcare Worker Education

2. All dental professionals must use surgical masks and protective eyewear to protect the eyes and face:
    c. In accordance with the Occupational Safety and Health Administration (OSHA)

Bloodborne Pathogens Standard, masks and protective eyewear are to be worn whenever splashes, spray, spatter, or droplets of blood or saliva may be generated and eye, nose, or mouth contamination may occur.
    CAT: Occupational Safety

3. All dental assistants involved in the direct provision of patient care must undergo routine training in:
    a. The Occupational Safety and Health Administration (OSHA) standard requires that employers shall ensure that all employees with occupational exposure participate in a training program on

the hazards associated with body fluids, protective measures to ensure safe practice, as well as hazard communications processes.
CAT: Patient and Dental Healthcare Worker Education

4. _____ occurs from a person previously contracting a disease and then recovering.
   a. When a microorganism invades the body, the body usually activates a special host defense system. Once this system is activated, it attempts to prevent serious harm from the microorganism and may provide protection against future invasions of the body by that same microorganism. This process is call naturally acquired immunity. Active natural immunity is when the host contracts a disease and produces antibodies that provide future resistance against that particular pathogen. Passive artificial immunity is received from an antiserum with antibodies from another host. Inherited immunity is present at birth.
   CAT: Patient and Dental Healthcare Worker Education

5. _____ immunity occurs when a vaccination is administered and the body forms antibodies in response to the vaccine.
   b. Active artificial immunity involves being immunized or vaccinated against a specific disease so that the body forms antibodies in response to the vaccine. Active natural immunity is when the host contracts a disease and produces antibodies that provide future resistance against that particular pathogen. Passive natural immunity is received through maternal antibodies form the placenta or breast milk. Passive artificial immunity is received from an antiserum with antibodies from another host.
   CAT: Patient and Dental Healthcare Worker Education

6. A latent infection is best exemplified by which of the following?
   b. A cold sore is a type of latent infection as it is quiet and inactive without manifesting itself until a period of incubation occurs. This is a persistent infection in which the

symptoms "come and go" unlike the other infections listed.
   CAT: Patient and Dental Healthcare Worker Education

7. Which of the following exemplifies an acute infection?
   c. An acute infection is one that has a rapid onset, severe symptoms, and a short course. The common cold is an example of such an infection. The other infections listed do not display these symptoms.
   CAT: Patient and Dental Healthcare Worker Education

8. Microorganisms that produce disease in humans are known as:
   b. A pathogen is a microorganism capable of causing disease in its host. An aerobe is a bacteria requiring oxygen to grow. Nonpathogenic is the opposite of pathogenic, and pasteurized does not relate to this statement.
   CAT: Patient and Dental Healthcare Worker Education

9. When should an alcohol hand rub be used for routine dentistry?
   c. Alcohol hand rubs may be used anytime but only when there is no visible soil on the hands.
   CAT: Preventing Cross-Contamination and Disease Transmission

10. An infection that occurs when the body's ability to resist diseases is weakened is:
    d. An opportunistic disease is one that will occur in the body when the person is unable to resist the infection or when the infection is given the opportunity.
    CAT: Patient and Dental Healthcare Worker Education

11. A disposable air/water syringe tip is to be:
    d. Disposable items are to be used only on one patient and then discarded.
    CAT: Preventing Cross-Contamination and Disease Transmission

12. The transmission of a disease through the skin, as with cuts or punctures, is _____ transmission.

b. Parenteral transmission of an infection refers to a mode of transmission that occurs through punctures or cuts in the skin.
CAT: Patient and Dental Healthcare Worker Education

13. Which of the following would be considered the best method for determining whether there is proper sterilization function by a sterilizer?
c. Biological monitoring or spore testing provides the main guarantee of sterilization accomplished by a sterilizer.
CAT: Instrument Processing

14. When leaving a patient at chairside to retrieve a supply item, which barrier should be removed and replaced after returning to the patient?
c. The gloves will be contaminated and would contaminate any surface touched when away from the patient unless the gloves are removed first.
CAT: Preventing Cross-Contamination and Disease Transmission

15. Protective eyewear should have:
c. Eyewear worn by the dental health care worker should have side shields to protect from aerosols and spatter.
CAT: Preventing Cross-Contamination and Disease Transmission

16. What is the most serious reaction to gloves?
c. Anaphylaxis can be life-threatening affecting breathing and blood flow. Dermatitis is a reaction to gloves but is not the most serious, and candidiasis is not a reaction to gloves.
CAT: Preventing Cross-Contamination and Disease Transmission

17. Which of the following is regulated medical waste?
c. All sharp contaminated items are considered as regulated medical waste and must be disposed of in appropriate containers.
CAT: Maintaining Aseptic Conditions

18. The microbes that contaminate the hands after touching surfaces are referred to as:
a. These microbes can be easily washed off the hands and are, therefore, referred to as transient.

CAT: Preventing Cross-Contamination and Disease Transmission

19. During which of the following procedures would you use sterile surgical gloves?
d. A mandibular resection is an invasive surgical procedure and would require the use of surgical gloves.
CAT: Preventing Cross-Contamination and Disease Transmission

20. Which of the following statements is an inappropriate action for postexposure medical evaluation and follow-up?
a. After the exposure incident, the employer must make immediately available to the exposed employee a medical evaluation performed by a licensed physician or other licensed health care professional at no cost to the employee.
CAT: Occupational Safety

21. Which of the following is a cause of sterilization failure?
c. A closed container prevents direct contact with the sterilizing agent.
CAT: Instrument Processing

22. To prevent contamination of surfaces, which of the following techniques should be used?
b. Applying covers after the surfaces become contaminated is a waste of money and time because the contaminated surfaces will have to be precleaned and disinfected when the patient leaves. The covers should be placed before the surfaces become contaminated and the cover should be carefully removed without touching the underlying surface. Covering surfaces is intended to replace precleaning and disinfecting between patients.
CAT: Asepsis Procedures

23. An emergency action plan may be communicated orally if the workplace has fewer than _____ employees.
d. According to the Fire Safety Standard of Occupational Safety and Health Administration (OSHA), an employer must review with each employee on initial assignment all parts of the fire safety plan that the employee must know to protect coworkers and patients in the event of an

emergency. For offices with fewer than 10 employees, the plan may be communicated orally, and the employer is not required to maintain a written plan.

CAT: Occupational Safety

24. What is the maximum volume that a single container of alcohol-based hand rub solution placed within a dental treatment room can legally have?

c. The American Society of Healthcare Engineering has issued a set of rules that include the placement of alcohol-based hand rubs. One of these rules states that single containers installed in the dental treatment room should not exceed a maximum capacity of 2.0 L of alcohol-based rub solutions in gel/liquid form.

CAT: Occupational Safety

25. Which of the following surfaces need not be cleaned and disinfected before each patient appointment?

b. Floors must be cleaned routinely but not after each patient. All of the other surfaces come into direct contact with patient care and must be cleaned and disinfected after each patient.

CAT: Asepsis Procedures

26. Which of the following is least important in protecting dental instruments?

d. Instruments are only dried before dry heat or chemical vapor sterilization to avoid corrosion aspects in these sterilizers.

CAT: Instrument Processing

27. Which of the following microbes on the hands are the most important in the spread of diseases?

a. The transient flora consists of microbes that are "picked up" by touching surfaces and are easily shed when other surfaces are touched.

CAT: Preventing Cross-Contamination and Disease Transmission

28. When alcohol hand rubs are used all day long why is it important to wash the hands every so often?

b. Since there is no rinsing associated with the use of alcohol hand rubs, gloves chemicals,

powder, and sweat accumulate on the hands and could cause some irritation.

CAT: Preventing Cross-Contamination and Disease Transmission

29. When should protective clothing be changed during the day?

a. Clothing is seldom involved in the spread of microbes except when it is visibly soiled.

CAT: Preventing Cross-Contamination and Disease Transmission

30. When an assistant transfers a microbe from one patient to his or her hand and then to another patient's mouth, this transmission is referred to as:

b. The mode of transmission where the disease results from injuries with contaminated sharps or from contact with contaminated hands, instruments, equipment, or surfaces is known as indirect contact.

CAT: Maintaining Aseptic Conditions

31. _____ is a protein manufactured in the body that binds to and destroys microbes and other antigens.

b. An antibody is a protein produced in response to an antigen that is capable of binding specifically to that antigen.

CAT: Patient and Dental Healthcare Worker Education

32. When should the surgical face mask be changed?

c. The outside of the mask becomes contaminated from spatter and handpiece sprays and by touching with contaminated gloved fingers. Thus the outside contamination may be spread to the next patient as one breaths or talks.

CAT: Preventing Cross-Contamination and Disease Transmission

33. What particles are involved in airborne transmission?

a. Airborne transmission involves the smallest particles such as aerosols. Spatter, droplets, and splashes are much larger than aerosol particles.

CAT: Preventing Cross-Contamination and Disease Transmission

34. Why should instruments be packaged before placing in a sterilizer?

b. Unpackaged instruments are immediately recontaminated when removed from the sterilizer through contact with materials in the air, on hands, and on surfaces.

CAT: **Maintaining Aseptic Conditions**

35. Recommendations concerning gloves would fall under which of the following categories of infection control practices that directly relate to dental radiography procedures?

b. Personal protective equipment (PPE) includes gloves, eyewear, and masks that are worn during routine clinical treatment to protect the dental health care worker.

CAT: **Preventing Cross-Contamination and Disease Transmission**

36. Protective clothing:

a. In accordance with Occupational Safety and Health Administration (OSHA) rules protective clothing must protect skin, work clothes, street clothes, and undergarments from exposure when contact with blood or other bodily fluids is anticipated.

CAT: **Preventing Cross-Contamination and Disease Transmission**

37. Amalgam contains which of the following hazardous materials?

c. Amalgam is used as a posterior filling material and contains mercury.

CAT: **Occupational Safety**

38. Special protective eyewear is to be worn when:

a. Some curing lights produce a wavelength that can be damaging to the eyes.

CAT: **Occupational Safety**

39. A latex allergy is caused by sensitivity to:

c. Proteins in the liquid latex "sap" collected from rubber trees serve as allergens to which some people are sensitive.

CAT: **Occupational Safety**

40. Which of the following best explains the relationship between latex allergies and glove powder (cornstarch)?

d. The powder adsorbs latex protein allergens from the gloves and when it becomes airborne it spreads the allergens around the office.

CAT: **Occupational Safety**

41. When using medical latex or vinyl gloves, _____.

b. Nonsterile gloves are recommended for routine dental care and nonsurgical procedures. Sterile gloves would be used in surgical or invasive procedures. Gloves are never rewashed or reused.

CAT: **Preventing Cross-Contamination and Disease Transmission**

42. _____ is defined as the absence of pathogens, or disease-causing microorganisms

d. The absence of infection or infectious materials or agents is known as the state of asepsis. An antiseptic is a substance used for killing microorganisms on the skin, and an antibiotic is a subgroup of antiinfectives that are derived from bacterial sources and are used to treat bacterial infections.

CAT: **Maintaining Aseptic Conditions**

43. Antiseptic refers to:

b. Antiseptics are chemical agents that can be used on external tissues to safely destroy microorganisms or to inhibit their growth.

CAT: **Maintaining Aseptic Conditions**

44. According to OSHA's Hazard Communication Standard the list of hazardous chemicals in the office needs to be cross-referenced to the:

b. If an exposure occurs, one can identify the chemical involved and locate the cross-referenced Material Safety Data Sheet that explains the hazards.

CAT: **Occupational Safety**

45. Which of the following agents is *not* tuberculocidal?

b. Quaternary ammonium compounds are categorized as low-level disinfectants and none are tuberculocidal.

CAT: **Asepsis Procedures**

46. When can a liquid sterilant/high-level disinfectant achieve sterilization?

b. High-level disinfectants can achieve sterilization when the solution is used only for longer exposure times in accordance with manufacturer's directions.

CAT: Instrument Processing

47. Which of the following may be used for surface disinfectant disinfection in the dental office?
    a. Most iodophors are intermediate-level disinfectants and can be used for surfaces in the treatment room. They do have a slightly corrosive effect to some metals and may cause a light staining if used repeatedly.
    CAT: Asepsis Procedures

48. Autoclaves are preset to reach a maximum steam temperature of ___ degrees Fahrenheit.
    c. Most manufacturers today preset the autoclave for steam under pressure sterilization to reach 250°F and pressure of 15 to 30 psi.
    CAT: Instrument Processing

49. The best way to avoid contracting a bloodborne disease in the office is to:
    c. Bloodborne diseases are spread by parenteral or mucous membrane contact with infected body fluids. Used sharps are usually contaminated with body fluids, and sharps injuries can "inject" such contaminates into the tissues.
    CAT: Occupational Safety

50. Which of the following is considered to be a semicritical instrument in radiography?
    d. The x-ray film-holding device is considered a semicritical rather than critical instrument, because it is not intended to penetrate tissue.
    CAT: Instrument Processing

51. Which of the following is a work practice control as described by OSHA?
    a. A work practice control alters the manner in which a task is performed to reduce the spread of contamination. This is in contrast to an engineering control which uses some type of equipment to reduce the spread of contamination.
    CAT: Occupational safety

52. Which method of sterilization requires good room ventilation?
    c. Unsaturated chemical vapor sterilization requires good room ventilation because the

active agent in the sterilizing solution used is formaldehyde.

CAT: Instrument Processing

53. OSHA requires which of the following documents to be present in every dental facility?
    c. A written exposure control plan that describes how employees will be protected from exposure to human body fluids is required by the Occupational Safety and Health Administration (OSHA) Bloodborne Pathogens Standard.
    CAT: Occupational Safety

54. Which government agency requires employers to protect their employees from exposure to blood and saliva at work?
    d. The Occupational Safety and Health Administration (OSHA) Bloodborne Pathogens Standard is the most important infection control law in dentistry to protect the dental health care workers.
    CAT: Occupational Safety

55. Improper cleaning or sterilizing of reusable hand instruments can contribute to which pathway of cross-contamination in the office?
    b. Patient-to-patient disease transmission is an indirect transfer of disease through improperly prepared instruments, handpieces and attachments, treatment room surfaces, and hands.
    CAT: Preventing Cross-Contamination and Disease Transmission

56. The main publication for all OSHA information is the:
    a. This is a daily publication from the federal government that includes information from the Occupational Safety and Health Administration (OSHA).
    CAT: Occupational Safety

57. From the list below, select the best procedure for caring for orthodontic wire.
    c. Orthodontic wire is defined as a sharp and is placed in the sharps container at the end of use.
    CAT: Maintaining Aseptic Conditions

58. From the list below, select the best procedure for caring for a pair of crown and collar scissors.

a. With sharp edges on the crown and collar scissors, the most efficient method of sterilization would be to place the scissors in a protective emulsion before placing in steam under pressure.
   CAT: Instrument Processing

59. From the list below, select the best procedure for caring for a pair of surgical suction tips.
   b. A surgical suction is used during an invasive procedure and the tip is generally made of metal and does not have any sharp edges. Therefore, it can be safely and efficiently placed in steam under pressure sterilization without the need to be placed in emulsion first.
   CAT: Instrument Processing

60. Which of the following is the recommended scheme for immunization against hepatitis B?
   a. The recommended scheme for immunization against hepatitis B for the dental health care worker is 0, 1, and 6 months.
   CAT: Occupational Safety

61. From the list below, select the best procedure for caring for a mandrel.
   b. A mandrel made of metal may be placed in steam under pressure without emulsion.
   CAT: Instrument Processing

62. The intent of handwashing is to remove:
   a. The microorganisms of transient skin flora contaminate the hands during the touching of or other exposure to contaminated surfaces. These flora serve as a source of disease spread because it can contain just about any pathogenic microorganism. Transient skin flora can be reduced or removed in some cases by routine handwashing because they remain primarily on the outer layers of the skin.
   CAT: Preventing Cross-Contamination and Disease Transmission

63. From the list below, select the best procedure for caring for a pair of protective glasses
   c. Protective eyewear cannot be subjected to heat and therefore must be disinfected.
   CAT: Asepsis Procedures

64. What is the active agent in hand rubs acceptable for use in dental offices?
   d. The agent in hand rubs used in the dental office is alcohol. It is used without water and without rinsing.
   CAT: Preventing Cross-Contamination and Disease Transmission

65. Which type of sterilization used in the dental office requires the longest processing time?
   c. Dry heat takes longer to sterilize than does steam under pressure or chemical vapor; it takes 1 hour at 320°F to 370°F depending on the type of sterilizer.
   CAT: Instrument Processing

66. What is required by the postexposure evaluation section of the Bloodborne Pathogens Standard?
   b. This standard requires employers to provide a postexposure medical evaluation to any employees who are exposed to human body fluids at work.
   CAT: Occupational Safety

67. Instruments have been in a liquid sterilant for 2 hours. The assistant adds another batch of instruments. Which of the following statements addresses this situation?
   d. Retiming must begin again when the second batch of instruments has been added to the original instruments that were immersed. The status of the original instruments has been altered, thus the retiming.
   CAT: Instrument Processing

68. According to the Bloodborne Pathogens Standard who must provide gloves, masks, eyeglasses, and protective clothing to the dental assistant in the office?
   b. The employer is required by the Occupational Safety and Health Administration (OSHA) to provide all the protective equipment needed to protect the employee from exposure to human body fluids.
   CAT: Occupational Safety

69. Which of the following methods of precleaning dental instruments should be avoided?
   c. Hand scrubbing is not a safe method for precleaning instruments. Instrument

washing machines, rinsing in a holding solution, and ultrasonic cleaning are the most efficient and safe modes of precleaning and cleaning instruments.

CAT: **Instrument Processing**

70. One of the main the purposes of the Hazard Communication Standard is to require:

    c. The Occupational Safety and Health Administration (OSHA) Hazard Communication Standard is designed to protect employees from exposure to hazardous chemical at work.

    CAT: **Occupational Safety**

71. Which of the following make laws that are associated with fines for noncompliance?

    b. The Occupational Safety and Health Administration (OSHA) makes laws while the Centers for Disease Control and Prevention (CDC), Organization for Safety, Asepsis and Prevention (OSAP), and the American Dental Association (ADA) make recommendations.

    CAT: **Occupational Safety**

72. The last of the PPEs to be put on before patient treatment begins is:

    c. Putting the gloves on last just before working on the patient's mouth limits the amount of contamination that is transferred to the patient.

    CAT: **Preventing Cross-Contamination and Disease Transmission**

73. Heavy utility gloves should be used:

    d. Heavy utility gloves give more protection to the hands than examination gloves when processing contaminated instruments.

    CAT: **Preventing Cross-Contamination and Disease Transmission**

74. Which of the following types of germicides can be used as a high-level disinfectant or a sterilant by following the manufacturer's guidelines for immersion time?

    b. Glutaraldehyde can serve as an immersion disinfectant at shorter exposure times (e.g., 30 minutes) and as a sterilant at longer exposure times (e.g., 3–10 hours).

    CAT: **Asepsis Procedures**

75. The 2012 update of the OSHA Hazard Communication Standard changed the name of Material Safety Data Sheets to:

    b. The phrase Safety Data Sheets is more in line with the Globally Harmonized System of Classification and Labeling of Chemicals to which the Occupational Safety and Health Administration (OSHA) is now related.

    CAT: **Occupational Safety**

76. The process that kills disease-causing microorganisms, but not necessarily all microbial life, is defined as:

    c. Disinfection destroys vegetative bacteria, some fungi, and some viruses; it does not destroy bacterial spores.

    CAT: **Asepsis Procedures**

77. The best way to determine that sterilization has actually occurred is to use:

    b. Biologic monitoring provides the most efficient guarantee of sterilization.

    CAT: **Instrument Processing**

78. The rule that requires employers to do certain things to prevent employees from being exposed to human body fluids at work is called the:

    d. This is an Occupational Safety and Health Administration (OSHA) standard that became effective in 1991.

    CAT: **Occupational Safety**

79. Patient care instruments are categorized into various classifications. Into which classification would instruments such as impression trays, dental mouth mirror, and amalgam condenser be placed?

    b. Impression trays, the dental mouth mirror, and the amalgam condenser are considered to be semicritical instruments because they are not intended to penetrate tissue.

    CAT: **Maintaining Aseptic Conditions**

80. Which of the following is least effective in minimizing the amount of dental aerosols and spatter generated during treatment?

    a. The amount of aerosols and spatter generated during dental treatment is not reduced by preprocedural mouth rinses. However, studies have shown that a mouth rinse with a long-lasting antimicrobial agent can reduce the level of oral microorganisms for up to 5 hours.

CAT: **Maintaining Aseptic Conditions**

81. Which of the following microbes will remain alive after exposure to an intermediate-level disinfectant?

    a. Intermediate-level disinfectants destroy vegetative bacteria, most fungi, and most viruses, as well as inactivate *Mycobacterium tuberculosis* var. *bovis* but they do not kill bacterial spores.

    CAT: **Asepsis Procedures**

82. Which of the following is the least appropriate PPE for cleaning and disinfecting a dental treatment room?

    c. For safe practice, latex examination gloves are not the personal protective equipment (PPE) of choice for cleaning and disinfecting a dental treatment room and its equipment. They give less protection to the hands than heavy utility gloves.

    CAT: **Asepsis Procedures**

83. The OSHA Bloodborne Pathogens Standard is designed to prevent which of the following diseases?

    c. Hepatitis C is one example of a bloodborne disease. Others are hepatitis B and D and human immunodeficiency virus (HIV).

    CAT: **Occupational Safety**

84. OSHA indicates that one way to prevent exposure to human body fluids is to use engineering controls. What is an engineering control?

    d. Examples of engineering controls include sharps containers, rubber dams, and high-volume evacuators.

    CAT: **Occupational Safety**

85. The Organization for Safety, Asepsis and Prevention identifies the classification of clinical touch surfaces to include which of the following?

    b. Clinical touch surfaces include light handles, dental unit controls, and chair switches, all items that are commonly touched during routine clinical treatment.

    CAT: **Asepsis Procedures**

86. Chemicals that destroy or inactivate most species of pathogenic microorganisms on inanimate surfaces are called:

    a. Disinfectants are used to destroy or inactivate most pathogenic microorganisms on inanimate surfaces such as countertops and flat cupboard surfaces.

    CAT: **Asepsis Procedures**

87. According to the OSHA Hazard Communication Standard, who determines the hazards of a chemical?

    c. The dental manufacturer is responsible for determining the hazards of a chemical and must provide an SDS for each product sent to the dental office.

    CAT: **Occupational Safety**

88. When a denture is to be repaired by a commercial laboratory, it should be:

    d. When a denture, other prosthesis, or an impression is sent to a commercial laboratory, it should be disinfected before being sent out and then again after being received back from the laboratory.

    CAT: **Asepsis Procedures**

89. A victim who feels the effects of a chemical spill immediately, with symptoms of dizziness, headache, nausea, and vomiting, is experiencing:

    b. When a person experiences an acute chemical toxicity, he or she will feel the effects immediately and will experience dizziness, headache, nausea, and vomiting.

    CAT: **Occupational Safety**

90. _____ is considered regulated waste and requires special disposal.

    a. Teeth and other waste tissues are considered potentially infectious, and thus their disposal is regulated.

    CAT: **Maintaining Aseptic Conditions**

91. The office safety supervisor should check the contents of the emergency kit to determine that the contents are in place and within the expiration date:

    b. First aid and emergency kits should be labeled and stored in an area easily accessible to the dental staff but out of sight

of patients. This kit should be checked each week to ensure currency.
CAT: Occupational Safety

92. Which of the following is to be used for cleaning and disinfecting blood-contaminated operatory surfaces?
    a. The Centers for disease Control and Prevention recommend that blood-contaminated surfaces be disinfected with an intermediate-level, rather than a low-level, disinfectant.
    CAT: Asepsis Procedures

93. All waste containers that hold potentially infectious materials must be:
    b. In accordance with the Occupational Safety and Health Administration (OSHA) regulations, all potentially infectious waste must be labeled with the biohazard symbol.
    CAT: Maintaining Aseptic Conditions

94. The OSHA Hazard Communications Standard requires employers to do all *except:*
    d. The Occupational Safety and Health Administration (OSHA) Hazard Communications Standard does not require employees to submit to an annual hair test.
    CAT: Occupational Safety

95. A dental health care worker transfers a small amount of cavity medication into a smaller container for use on a patient at chairside. A new label must be placed on that container if:
    b. When it is necessary to transfer a small amount of cavity medication from a large container into a smaller one, the new container must be labeled if it is not used up at the end of an 8-hour work day.
    CAT: Occupational Safety

96. The microbial accumulation on the inside walls of dental unit waterlines is best referred to as:
    b. A biofilm is a mass of microbes attached to a surface. Another example of a biofilm is dental plaque.
    CAT: Asepsis Procedures

97. The ADA, OSAP, and CDC recommend that the dental assistant:
    b. Various agencies, including American Dental Association (ADA), Organization for Safety, Asepsis and Prevention (OSAP), and Centers for Disease Control and Prevention (CDC), recommend that the dental assistant flush the dental unit waterlines for 20 to 30 seconds each morning and after each patient.
    CAT: Asepsis Procedures

98. For instruments to be sterilized, they must first be:
    b. For sterilization to be achieved, instruments must be free of blood or bioburden, which could prevent steam, unsaturated chemical vapor, or heat from directly contacting the instrument surfaces.
    CAT: Instrument Processing

99. Who is required by the Occupational Safety and Health Administration to pay for the protective clothing used by dental assistants?
    b. The Occupational Safety and Health Administration (OSHA) Bloodborne Pathogens Standard states that the employer must provide all personal protective equipment (PPE) for employees who may become exposed to patients' body fluids.
    CAT: Occupational Safety

100. According to the Occupational Safety and Health Administration (OSHA), who pays for the OSHA-required training for employees in the dental office?
    a. The Bloodborne Pathogens Standard states that the employer must provide specific ·training for employees who may become exposed to patients' body fluids.
    CAT: Occupational Safety

Contacts

NATIONAL CONTACTS

American Dental Association
211 East Chicago Avenue
Chicago, Illinois 60611-2678
312-440-2500
www.ada.org

American Dental Assistants Association
35 East Wacker Drive
Suite 1730
Chicago, Illinois 60601-2211
312-541-1550
www.dentalassistant.org

The Dental Assisting National Board, Inc. (DANB)
444 North Michigan Avenue
Suite 900
Chicago, Illinois 60611-3985
1-800-367-3262 or 312-642-3368
www.danb.org

STATE CONTACTS

Board of Dental Examiners of Alabama
www.dentalboard.org
205-985-7267

Alaska State Board of Dental Examiners
www.dced.state.ak.us/occ/pden.htm
907-465-2542

Arizona State Board of Dental Examiners
www.azdentalboard.org
602-242-1492

Arkansas State Board of Dental Examiners
www.asbde.org
501-682-2085

Dental Board of California
http://www.dbc.ca.gov/
(916) 263-2300

Colorado State Board of Dental Examiners
www.dora.state.co.us/dental
303-894-7758

Connecticut State Dental Commission/
  Department of Public Health
www.dph.state.ct.us/bch/oralhealth/index
860-509-8388

Delaware Department of Health
www.dpr.delaware.gov/boards/dental/index.shtml
302-744-4700

Department of Health-District of Columbia
  Board of Dentistry
http://doh.dc.gov/
202-724-4900

Florida Board of Dentistry
www.doh.state.fl.us/mqa/dentistry/
850-245-4474

Georgia Board of Dentistry
www.sos.state.ga.us/plb/dentistry
478-207-2445

Hawaii State Board of Dental Examiners
www.hawaii.gov/dcca/areas/pvl/boards/dentist
808-586-3000

Idaho State Board of Dentistry
http://isbd.idaho.gov/
208-334-2369

Illinois State Board of Dentistry
www.idfpr.com
217-782-8556

Indiana State Department of Health
http://www.state.in.us/isdh/
317-233-7565

Iowa Board of Dental Examiners
www.state.ia.us/dentalboard
515-281-5157

Kansas Dental Board
www.accesskansas.org/kdb
785-296-6400

Kentucky Board of Dentistry
www.dentistry.ky.gov
502-429-7280

Louisiana State Board of Dentistry
www.lsbd.org
504-568-8574

Maine Board of Dental Examiners
www.mainedental.org
207-287-3333

Maryland State Board of Dental Examiners
www.dhmh.state.md.us/dental
410-402-8500

Massachusetts Board of Registration in Dentistry
www.mass.gov/dpl/boards/dn
617-973-0971

Michigan Board of Dentistry
www.michigan.gov/healthlicense
517-335-0918

Minnesota Board of Dentistry
www.dentalboard.state.mn.us
612-617-2250

Mississippi State Board of Dental Examiners
www.msbde.state.ms.us
601-944-9622

Missouri Dental Board
pr.mo.gov/dental.asp
573-751-0040

Montana Board of Dentistry
www.discoveringmontana.com/dli/den
406-841-2390

Nebraska Board of Dentistry – Credentialing Division
http://dhhs.ne.gov/publichealth/Pages/public_health_index.aspx
402-471-2118

Nevada State Board of Dental Examiners
http://www.nvdentalboard.nv.gov/
1-800-DDS-EXAM or 702-486-7044

New Hampshire Board of Dental Examiners
www.state.nh.us/dental
603-271-4561

New Jersey State Board of Dentistry
www.state.nj.us/lps/ca/medical/dentistry.htm
973-504-6405

New Mexico Board of Dental Health Care
http://www.rld.state.nm.us/boards/Dental_Health_Care.aspx
505-476-4680

New York State Board for Dentistry
http://www.op.nysed.gov/prof/dent/
518-474-3817

North Carolina State Board of Dental Examiners
www.ncdentalboard.org
919-678-8223

North Dakota State Board of Dental Examiners
www.nddentalboard.org
701-258-8600

Ohio State Dental Board
www.dental.ohio.gov
614-466-2580

Oklahoma State Board of Dentistry
http://www.boardofdentistry.net/oklahoma-board-of-dentistry
405-524-9037

Oregon Board of Dentistry
www.oregondentistry.org
503-229-5520

Pennsylvania State Board of Dentistry
www.dos.state.pa.us/dent
717-783-7162

Rhode Island State Board of Examiners in Dentistry
www.health.ri.gov/hsr/professions/dental.php
401-222-1392

South Carolina State Board of Dentistry
http://www.llr.state.sc.us/pol/dentistry/
803-896-4599

South Dakota State Board of Dentistry
www.state.sd.us/doh/dentistry
605-224-1282

Tennessee Board of Dentistry
http://health.state.tn.us/Boards/Dentistry
800-778-4123 x24721

Texas State Board of Dental Examiners
www.tsbde.state.tx.us
512-463-6400

Utah Dentists and Dental Hygienists
   Licensing Board
www.dopl.utah.gov/licensing/dentistry.html
801-530-6740

Vermont State Board of Dental Examiners
www.vtprofessionals.org/opr1/dentists
802-828-2390

Virginia Board of Dentistry
www.dhp.virginia.gov/dentistry/default.htm
804-662-9906

Washington State Dental Health Care Authority
http://www.hca.wa.gov/about.html
360-236-4822

West Virginia Board of Dental Examiners
www.wvdentalboard.org
877-914-8266

Wisconsin Dentistry Examining Board
drl.wi.gov/boards/den/index.htm
608-266-2811

Wyoming Board of Dental Examiners
plboards.state.wy.us/dental/index.asp
307-777-6529

Bibliography/ Suggested Readings

Listed below is a series of references used as resources to create the examinations. You may find it helpful to review these books as you proceed to prepare for a credentialing exam or to use for future reference:

1. Anusavice KJ: *Psillips' Science of Dental Materials*, ed 12, St. Louis, 2013, Saunders.
2. Chiego DJ: *Essentials of Oral Histology and Embryology: A Clinical Approach*, ed 4, St. Louis, 2014, Mosby.
3. Beemsterboer PL: *Ethics and Law in Dental Hygiene*, ed 2, St. Louis, 2010, Saunders.
4. Bennett J, Rosenberg M: *Medical Emergencies in Dentistry*, St. Louis, 2002, Saunders.
5. Bird DL, Robinson DS: *Modern Dental Assisting*, ed 11, St. Louis, 2015, Saunders.
6. Boyd LB: *Dental Instruments: A Pocket Guide*, ed 5, St. Louis, 2015, Saunders.
7. Brand RW, Isselhard DE: *Anatomy of Orofacial Structures*, ed 7 (enhanced), St. Louis, 2014, Elsevier.
8. Burt BA, Eklund SA: *Dentistry, Dental Practice and the Community*, ed 6, St. Louis, 2005, Saunders.
9. Cappelli DP, Mobley CC: *Prevention in Clinical Oral Health Care*, St. Louis, 2008, Mosby.
10. Centers for Disease Control and Prevention, Guidelines for Infection Control in Dental Healthcare Settings – 2003, *MMWR* 52(RR-17):1–68, 2003. also available at: www.cdc.gov/mmwr/PDF/rr/rr5217.pdf.
11. *Centers for Disease Control and Prevention and the Healthcare Infection Control Practices Advisory Committee (HICPAC), Guidelines for Environmental Infection Control in Healthcare Facilities* available at: www.cdc.gov/ncidod/dhqp/gl_environinfection.html.
12. Clark M, Brunick A: *Handbook of Nitrous Oxide and Oxygen Sedation*, ed 4, St. Louis, 2015, Mosby.
13. *DANB GC Review Part I,* Chicago, 2011 (updated 2015), The DALE Foundation.
14. *DANB GC Practice Test,* Chicago, 2012, The DALE Foundation.
15. *DANB GC Review Part II,* Chicago, 2011 (updated 2015), The DALE Foundation.
16. *DANB ICE Practice Test,* Chicago, 2012, The DALE Foundation.
17. *DANB ICE Review,* Chicago, 2011 (updated 2014), The DALE Foundation.
18. *DANB RHS Practice Test,* Chicago, 2011, The DALE Foundation.
19. *DANB RHS Review,* Chicago, 2010 (updated 2013), The DALE Foundation.
20. Daniel SJ, Harfst SAC, Wilder R: *Mosby's Dental Hygiene: Concepts, Cases and Competencies*, ed 2, St. Louis, 2008, Mosby.
21. Darby ML: *Mosby's Comprehensive Review of Dental Hygiene*, ed 7, St. Louis, 2012, Mosby.
22. Darby ML, Walsh M: *Dental Hygiene Theory and Practice*, ed 4, St. Louis, 2015, Saunders.
23. Davison JA: *Legal and Ethical Considerations for Dental Hygienists and Assistants*, St. Louis, 2000, Mosby.
24. Elsevier: *Legal and Ethical Issues for Health Professions,* ed 3, St. Louis, 2015, Elsevier.
25. Fehrenbach MJ, Herring SW: *Illustrated Anatomy of the Head and Neck*, ed 4, St. Louis, 2012, Saunders.
26. Fehrenbach MJ, Popowics T: *Illustrated Dental Embryology, Histology, and Anatomy*, ed 4, St. Louis, 2016, Elsevier.
27. Fehrenbach MJ, Weiner J: *Saunders Review of Dental Hygiene*, ed 2, St. Louis, 2009, Saunders.
28. Finkbeiner BL, Finkbeiner CA: *Practice Management for the Dental Team*, ed 8, St. Louis, 2016, Mosby.
29. Finkbeiner BL, Johnson CS: *Mosby's Comprehensive Review of Dental Assisting*, St. Louis, 1997, Mosby.
30. Frommer HH, Stabulas-Savage JJ: *Radiology for the Dental Professional*, ed 9, St. Louis, 2010, Mosby.
31. Gaylor L: *The Administrative Dental Assistant*, ed 3, St. Louis, 2012, Saunders.
32. Gluck GM, Morganstein WM: *Jong's Community Dental Health*, ed 5, St. Louis, 2002, Mosby.
33. Guerink KV: *Community Oral Health Practice for the Dental Hygienist*, ed 3, St. Louis, 2012, Saunders.
34. Hatrick CD, Eakle S: *Dental Materials: Clinical Applications for Dental Assistants and Dental Hygienists*, ed 3, Philadelphia, 2016, Saunders.
35. Haveles EB: *Applied Pharmacology for the Dental Hygienist*, ed 7, St. Louis, 2016, Mosby.
36. Hupp JR, Williams T, Firriolo FJ: *Dental Clinical Advisor*, St. Louis, 2006, Mosby.
37. Iannucci JM, Howerton LJ: *Dental Radiography: Principles and Techniques*, ed 4, St. Louis, 2012, Saunders.
38. Ibsen OAC, Phelan JA: *Oral Pathology for the Dental Hygienist*, ed 6, St. Louis, 2014, Saunders.
39. Langlais RP: *Exercises in Oral Radiology and Interpretation*, ed 4, St. Louis, 2004, Saunders.

40. Little JW, Falace D, Miller CS, Rhodus NL: *Dental Management of the Medically Compromised Patient*, ed 7, St. Louis, 2013, Mosby.

41. Malamed SF: *Sedation: A Guide to Patient Management*, ed 5, St. Louis, 2010, Mosby.

42. Malamed SF: *Medical Emergencies in the Dental Office*, ed 7, St. Louis, 2015, Mosby.

43. Miller CH: *Infection Control & Management of Hazardous Materials for the Dental Team*, ed 5, St. Louis, 2014, Mosby.

44. Mosby: *Spanish Terminology for the Dental Team*, ed 2, St. Louis, 2011, Mosby.

45. Mosby: *Mosby's Dental Dictionary*, ed 3, St. Louis, 2014, Mosby.

46. Mosby, Jeske AH: *Mosby's Dental Drug Reference*, ed 11, St. Louis, 2014, Mosby.

47. Nanci A: *Ten Cate's Oral Histology: Development, Structure and Function*, ed 8, St. Louis, 2013, Mosby.

48. Nelson SJ: *Wheeler's Dental Anatomy, Physiology, & Occlusion*, ed 10, St. Louis, 2015, Elsevier.

49. Neville BW, Damm DD, Allen CM, Chi AC: *Oral and Maxillofacial Pathology*, ed 4, St. Louis, 2016, Saunders.

50. Newman MG, Takei H, Klokkevold PR, Carranza FA: *Carranza's Clinical Periodontology*, ed 12, St. Louis, 2015, Saunders.

51. Organization for Safety and Aseptic Procedures: *From Policy to Practice: OSAP's Guide to the Guidelines*, Annapolis, 2004, OSAP.

52. Perry DA, Beemsterboer PL, Essex G: *Periodontology for the Dental Hygienist*, ed 4, St. Louis, 2014, Saunders.

53. Powers JM, Wataha JC: *Dental Materials: Properties and Manipulation*, ed 10, St. Louis, 2013, Mosby.

54. Regezi JA, Sciubba JJ, Jordan RCK: *Oral Pathology: Clinical Pathologic Correlations*, ed 6, St. Louis, 2012, Saunders.

55. Robinson DS, Bird DL: *Essentials of Dental Assisting*, ed 5, St. Louis, 2013, Elsevier.

56. Samaranayake LP: *Essential Microbiology for Dentistry*, ed 4, St. Louis, 2012, Saunders.

57. Stegeman CA, Davis JR: *The Dental Hygienist's Guide to Nutritional Care*, ed 4, St. Louis, 2015, Saunders.

58. United States Department of Labor, Occupational Safety and Health Administration, 29 CFR Part 1910.1030. Occupational Exposure to Bloodborne Pathogens; Needlesticks and Other Sharps Injuries; Final Rule, *Federal Register* 66:5317–5325, 2001. As amended from and includes 29 CFR Part 1910.1030. Occupational Exposure to Bloodborne Pathogens; Final Rule. *Federal Register* 1991; 56:64174–82, available at www.osha.gov/SLTC/dentistry/index.html.

59. United States Department of Labor, Occupational Safety and Health Administration, 29 CFR 1910.1030. Hazard Communications; Final Rule, *Federal Register* 59:6126–6184, 1994, also available at: www.osha.gov/SLTC/hazardcommunications/index.html.

Figure Credits

Test 1 General Chairside

Figures corresponding to questions 58, 64, 69, 80, 81 from Bird DL and Robinson DS: *Modern Dental Assisting,* ed 10, St. Louis, 2012, Saunders.

Figures corresponding to questions 86 and 87, courtesy of Miltex, Inc, York, Pennsylvania.

Test 1 Radiation Health and Safety

Figures corresponding to questions 12, 36, 99, and 100 from Iannucci JM, Howerton LJ: *Dental Radiography: Principles and Techniques,* ed 4, St. Louis, 2012, Saunders.

Test 2 General Chairside

Figures corresponding to questions 14–20 from Bird DL and Robinson DS: *Modern Dental Assisting,* ed 10, St. Louis, 2012, Saunders.

Figure corresponding to question 37 from Finkbeiner B and Johnson C: *Mosby's Comprehensive Dental Assisting: A Clinical Approach,* St. Louis, 1995, Mosby.

Figures corresponding to questions 44, 45, 50, 79 from Boyd LB: *Dental Instruments: A Pocket Guide,* ed 4, St. Louis, 2012, Saunders.

Test 2 Radiation Health and Safety

Figures corresponding to questions 10, 11, 12, and 100 from Iannucci JM, Howerton LJ: *Dental Radiography: Principles and Techniques,* ed 4, St. Louis, 2012, Saunders.

Test 3 General Chairside

Figure corresponding to question 18 from Finkbeiner B and Johnson C: *Mosby's Comprehensive Dental Assisting: A Clinical Approach,* St. Louis, 1995, Mosby.

Figures corresponding to questions 24 from Boyd LB: *Dental Instruments: A Pocket Guide,* ed 4, St. Louis, 2012, Saunders.

Figures corresponding to questions 5, 6, 9-12, 31, 32, 44 from Bird DL and Robinson DS: *Modern Dental Assisting,* ed 10, St. Louis, 2012, Saunders.

Test 3 Radiation Health and Safety

Figures corresponding to questions 8, 10, 13, 15, and 100 from Iannucci JM, Howerton LJ: *Dental Radiography: Principles and Techniques,* ed 4, St. Louis, 2012, Saunders.